Wall Pilates Workouts For Women

Step-by-step illustrated guides to improve posture and muscle tone, abs and hips

By

Rylan Stone

Contents

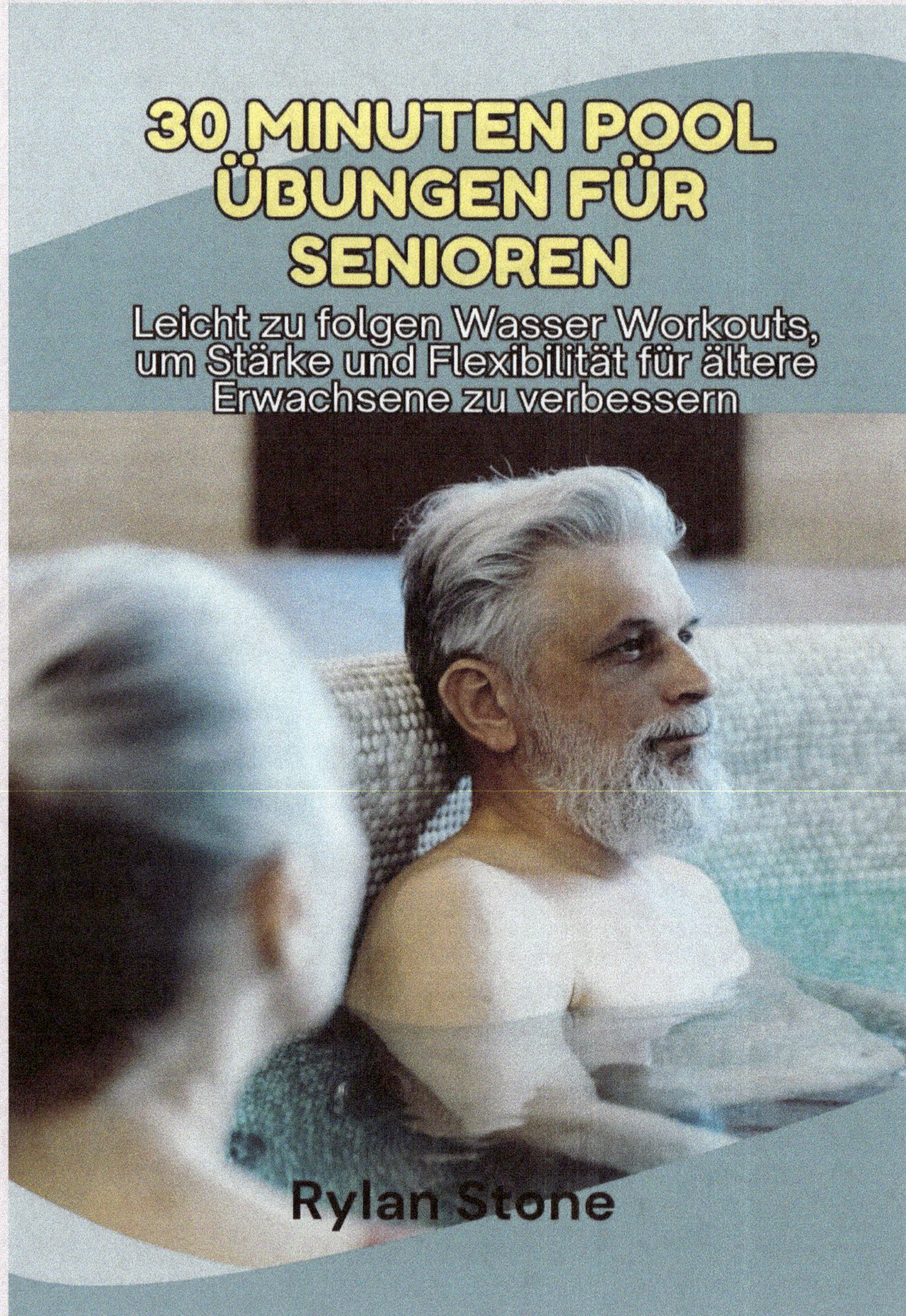
30 MINUTEN POOL ÜBUNGEN FÜR SENIOREN
Leicht zu folgen Wasser Workouts, um Stärke und Flexibilität für ältere Erwachsene zu verbessern
Rylan Stone

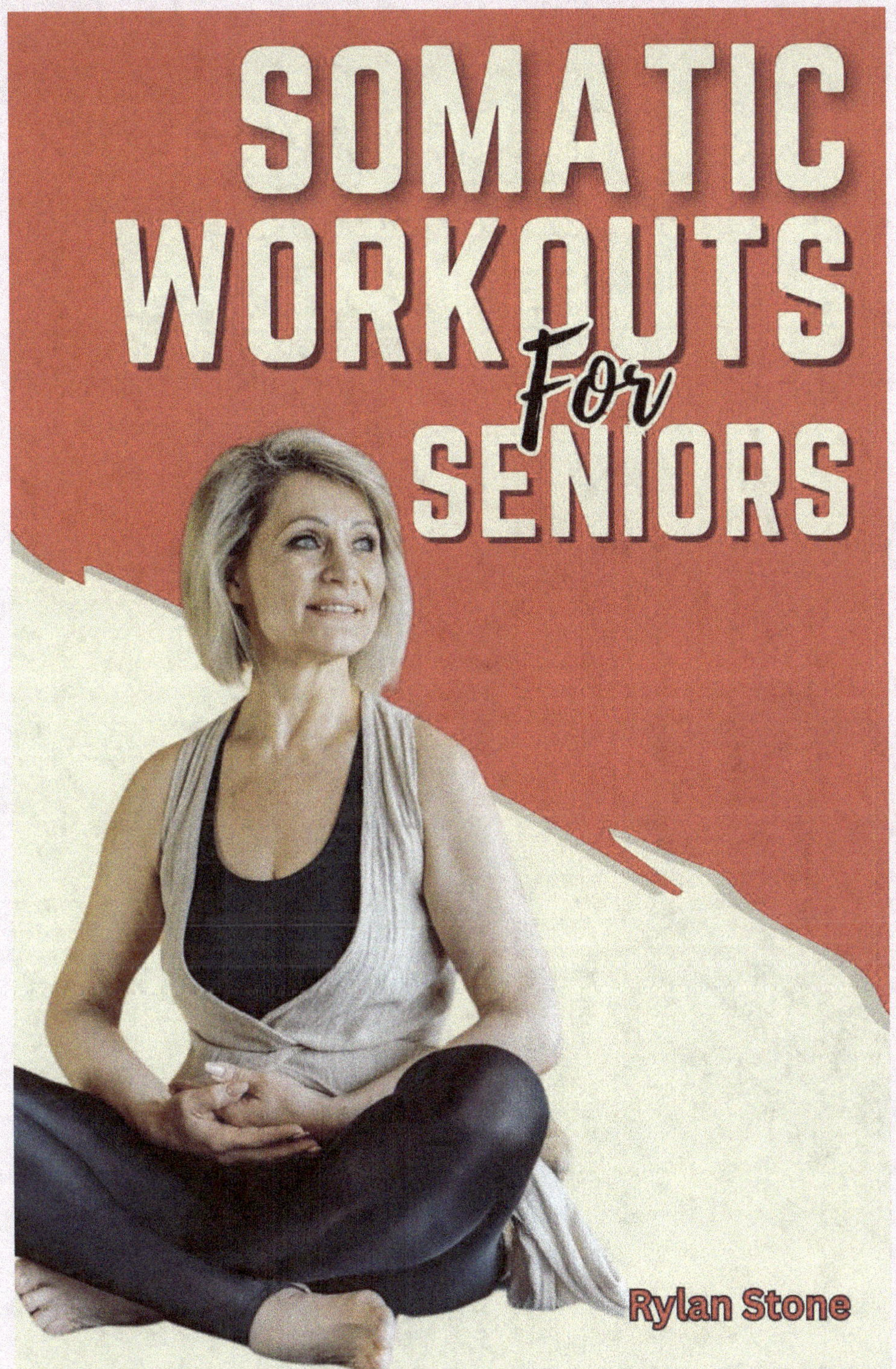
SOMATIC
WORKOUTS
For
SENIORS
Rylan Stone

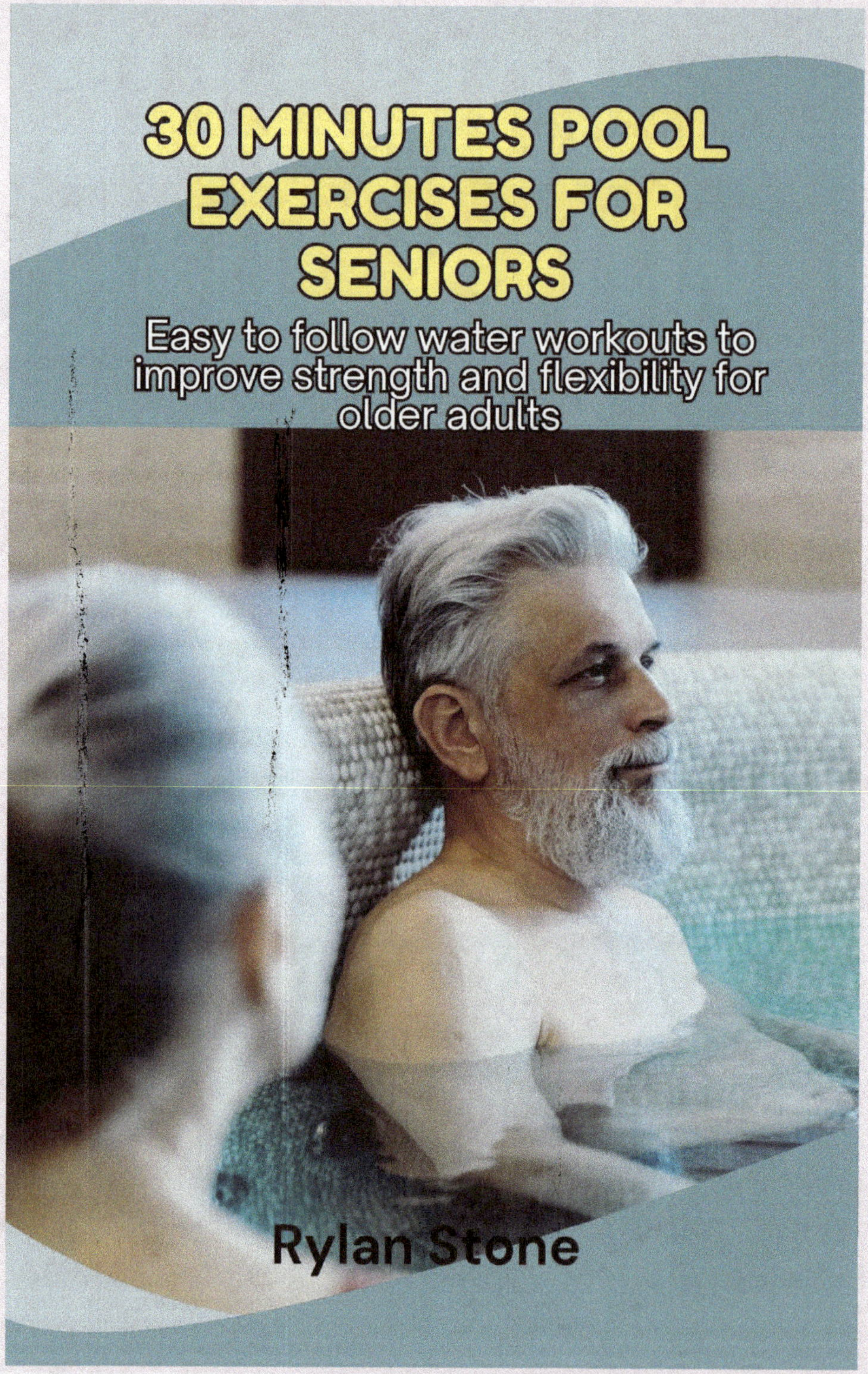

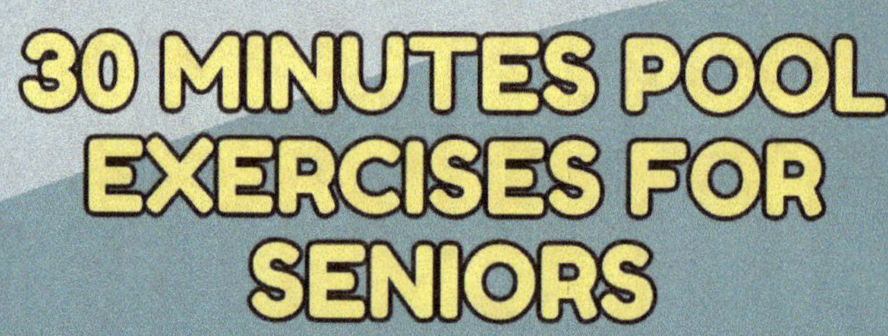

30 MINUTES POOL EXERCISES FOR SENIORS

Easy to follow water workouts to improve strength and flexibility for older adults

Rylan Stone

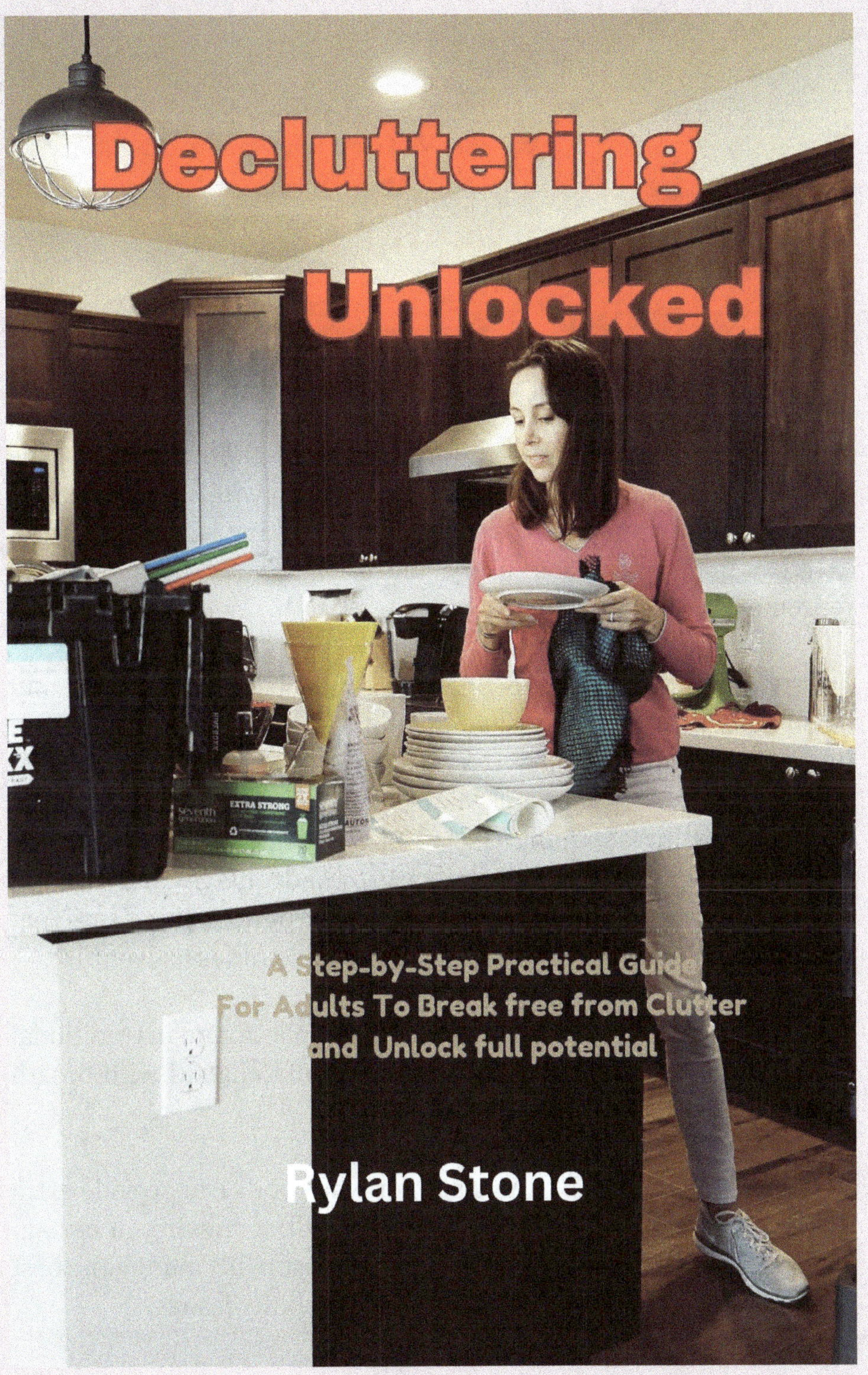
Decluttering
Unlocked
A Step-by-Step Practical Guide
For Adults To Break free from Clutter
and Unlock full potential
Rylan Stone

Chapter 1

Introduction to Wall Pilates

Wall Pilates is a smart choice for alternative and more accessible form of the traditional workout, providing you with an entirely new way to achieve your fitness goals if youre looking for a low-impact exercise that will reach every muscle on your body even in retirement age.

This type of practice allows people to build balance, strength and flexibility with the support and stability of a wall as a prop, which significantly reduces injury.

Through this introduction to Wall Pilates, we'll help you discover the key principles of learning it, its various advantages and how can it be combined with your somatic workout around making sure that our consumers have a complete and enjoyable fitness adventure.

Wall Pilates incorporates many of the principles found in traditional Pilates practices, such as specific movements aligned with breath control and utilizing core strength.

Using the wall as a prop to help support your body can provide extra stability and support for those with difficulties moving in certain ways or concerns about balance. For this reason, it's among the best yoga poses to do using a wall if you have mobility issues.

Benefits Of Wall Pilates

Balance and stability are one of the major advantages of Wall Pilates. "The older we get, the more we need to make sure that these primary aspects of fitness are addressed because this can save us from some nasty falls and injuries," he adds. Doing Pilates exercises along a wall can help to increase your sense of balance in a relatively secure manner, allowing you to gain the confidence that it will take for you to become more stable.

Another benefit of Wall Pilates is the promotion of strength and flexibility. Lean muscle mass is built using your body weight as resistance, and joint mobility and range of motion are also increased. In addition, Wall Pilates promotes proper posture and body alignment. Improved posture can aid in the reduction of chronic pain and the avoidance of musculoskeletal disorders.

Wall Pilates is a natural complement to your somatic program. Somatics and Pilates can easily be combined because both disciplines emphasize mindful movement via breath control and physical consciousness. Wall Pilates is a wonderful way to refresh your experience and create a fitness regimen that supports overall wellness.

Wall Pilates provides a secure, efficient, and pleasurable method for older individuals to improve their stability, power, and agility, all while adopting a mindful approach to physical fitness. By integrating this exercise into your somatic workout regimen, you can establish a holistic and personalized fitness journey that promotes your overall health and happiness during your years.

Importance of Wall Pilates for women's health and wellness

Pelvic Floor Health:

Wall Pilates includes exercises that specifically focus on the muscles of the pelvic floor. These muscles play a crucial role in maintaining control over urinary functions, sexual function, and overall core stability. Strengthening these muscles is especially important for women, particularly after giving birth or during menopause, as these life stages can bring about pelvic floor issues.

Bone Health:

Women have a higher likelihood of developing osteoporosis, especially after going through menopause. Wall Pilates offers a safe and effective way to engage in weight-bearing exercises, which are known to help maintain and enhance bone density. By doing so, the risk of fractures and osteoporosis can be significantly reduced.

hormone regulation:

engaging in regular exercises, such as wall pilates, can assist in the regulation of hormones, which is particularly crucial for women who experience hormonal changes during menstruation, pregnancy, or menopause. maintaining balanced hormone levels contributes to overall health, stability in mood, and a decreased risk of health issues related to hormones.

stress management:

women often find themselves juggling various responsibilities, leading to stress and anxiety. the focus on mindfulness and breath control in wall pilates helps promote relaxation and relief from stress, fostering a more harmonious state of mind and overall well-being.

body confidence and self-esteem:

participating in regular physical activity, like wall pilates, can enhance body image and self-esteem. As women progress in their practice and witness improvements in strength, flexibility, and balance, they develop a greater appreciation for their bodies and their capabilities.

Chapter 2

Understanding Your Body

This involves learning how to move your body in a way that is safe and effective, minimizing the risk of injury and maximizing the benefits of your workout. By focusing on proper alignment, posture, and movement mechanics, you can ensure that you are engaging the correct muscles and joints, and avoid putting unnecessary strain on your body.

In addition to physical awareness, the somatic workout also emphasizes the importance of mental and emotional awareness. By being present in the moment and tuning into your thoughts and emotions during exercise, you can develop a deeper connection between your mind and body. This mind-body connection not only enhances the effectiveness of your workout but also promotes overall well-being and stress reduction.

Ultimately, the somatic workout is about developing a holistic understanding of your body and treating it with respect and care. By prioritizing mindful movement, self-awareness, and personalized fitness routines, you can create a sustainable and enjoyable fitness journey that supports your unique needs and goals.

By placing more importance on the quality of your movements rather than the quantity, you can reduce the chances of getting injured and ensure that each movement is effective and safe. This approach promotes being mindful and establishes a stronger connection between your mind and body.

Understanding your body also involves adapting your somatic workout to accommodate any physical limitations or health concerns. This means modifying exercises and adjusting the intensity or complexity of your fitness routine, so you can still enjoy the benefits of physical activity while respecting your body's limitations.

To maintain overall health and well-being, it is crucial to incorporate restorative practices into your fitness routine. This can include gentle stretching, relaxation techniques, or meditation. Prioritizing recovery and giving your body time to heal and rejuvenate will support your long-term fitness goals and help you achieve a balanced lifestyle.

Summary of the female physique and its distinct requirements

The female body has distinct characteristics and needs that differ from those of the male body. Here is a summary of the specific requirements of the female body:

1. Hormonal differences: Women have higher levels of estrogen and progesterone, which impact body composition, metabolism, and muscle growth.

2. Body composition: Women generally have a higher proportion of body fat, especially in the hips, thighs, and buttocks.

3. Pelvic structure: Women have a wider pelvis and a larger Q-angle, which affects knee alignment and movement.

4. Muscle development: Women typically have less muscle mass and strength compared to men, particularly in the upper body.

5. Core stability: Women have a deeper pelvis and a more flexible spine, necessitating a greater focus on core stability and activation.

6. Women generally have greater flexibility and range of motion, especially in the hips and pelvis.

7. The changes that occur in a woman's body during pregnancy and childbirth significantly affect the pelvic floor, core, and overall physical functioning.

8. The monthly hormonal fluctuations that women experience during their menstrual cycle can impact their energy levels, mood, and physical performance.

9. Women are more prone to experiencing changes in bone density, such as osteoporosis, especially after menopause.

10. Women have specific nutritional needs, including higher requirements for iron and calcium, and are more susceptible to dehydration.

These unique physiological and hormonal characteristics of women require customized approaches to fitness, nutrition, and overall well-being.

Understanding your core, posture, and alignment

core:

- The core encompasses the muscles in your midsection, such as your abs, obliques, and lower back muscles.
- A strong core provides stability and support for your entire body.

- When practicing wall pilates, engaging your core muscles helps maintain proper posture, balance, and control during exercises.

posture:

- Maintaining good posture involves keeping your spine in a neutral alignment, with your ears, hips, knees, and ankles all in line.
- Wall pilates helps improve posture by strengthening the muscles that support the spine and promoting awareness of proper alignment.
- Women often find focusing on posture beneficial to counteract the impact of pregnancy, childbirth, and menopause on the spine and pelvis.

alignment:

- Alignment refers to how your body is positioned between the wall and the floor.

- In wall pilates, proper alignment ensures that you are targeting the correct muscles and avoiding unnecessary strain on your joints.

Women should concentrate on keeping their pelvis in a neutral position, activating their core muscles, and ensuring that their shoulders are relaxed and not hunched up towards their ears.

By paying attention to these aspects during Wall Pilates workouts, women can achieve various benefits such as enhancing their overall core strength and stability, improving their posture and reducing back pain, increasing their flexibility and mobility, promoting pelvic floor health and stability, and boosting their confidence and overall well-being.

Identifying and addressing common areas of tension and weakness

Identifying and addressing common areas of tension and weakness is crucial for women's overall health and well-being, especially when it comes to Wall Pilates workouts.

1. **Neck and Shoulders:**
   - Tension can arise from stress, bad posture, and excessive computer use.
   - Weakness can be found in the shoulder blades and upper back muscles.

2. **Upper Back and Thoracic Spine:**
   - Tension can be caused by poor posture, heavy breasts, and bra straps.
   - Weakness can be found in the mid-back muscles and flexibility of the thoracic spine.

3. **Lower Back and Pelvis:**
   - Tension can arise from pregnancy, childbirth, and menopause.
   - Weakness can be found in the core muscles, pelvic floor, and gluteal muscles.

4. **Hips and Glutes:**
   - Tension can be caused by prolonged sitting, poor posture, and hormonal changes.
   - Weakness can be found in the gluteal muscles and flexibility of the hips.

5. **Knees and Ankles:**
   - Tension can arise from wearing high heels, improper footwear, and overuse.

- Weakness can be found in ankle stability and proper alignment of the knees.

To address these areas, incorporate the following Wall Pilates exercises and tips:

1. **Neck and Shoulders:**
   - Perform the Chest Expansion exercise by standing with feet shoulder-width apart and extending the arms while pressing the chest forward.
   - Do Shoulder Rolls by rolling the shoulders forward and backward in a circular motion.

2. **Upper Back and Thoracic Spine:**
   - Perform the Cat-Cow exercise to flex and extend the spine, focusing on improving mobility in the middle of the back.
   - Engage the shoulder blades by squeezing them together and hold for 5 seconds.

3. **Lower Back and Pelvis:**
   - Tilt the pelvis up and back to engage the core muscles with the Pelvic Tilt exercise.
   - Strengthen the gluteal muscles by folding the knees while keeping the feet flat on the ground.

4. **Hips and Glutes:**
   - Target the gluteal muscles by lifting the legs out to the sides with Side Leg Lifts.
   - Move the hips in a large circular motion, first clockwise and then counterclockwise, with Hip Circles.

5. **Knees and Ankles:**
   - Improve ankle mobility by rotating the ankles in a circular motion, first clockwise and then counterclockwise, with Ankle Mobilization.

- Strengthen the quadriceps by straightening the knees while keeping the feet flat on the ground with Knee Extensions.

Remember to:
- Start slowly and gradually increase intensity.
- Engage the core muscles and maintain proper alignment.
- Breathe naturally and smoothly.
- Listen to your body and modify or rest when necessary.

By addressing these common areas of tension and weakness, women can enhance overall strength, flexibility, and posture, reducing the risk of injury and improving overall well-being.

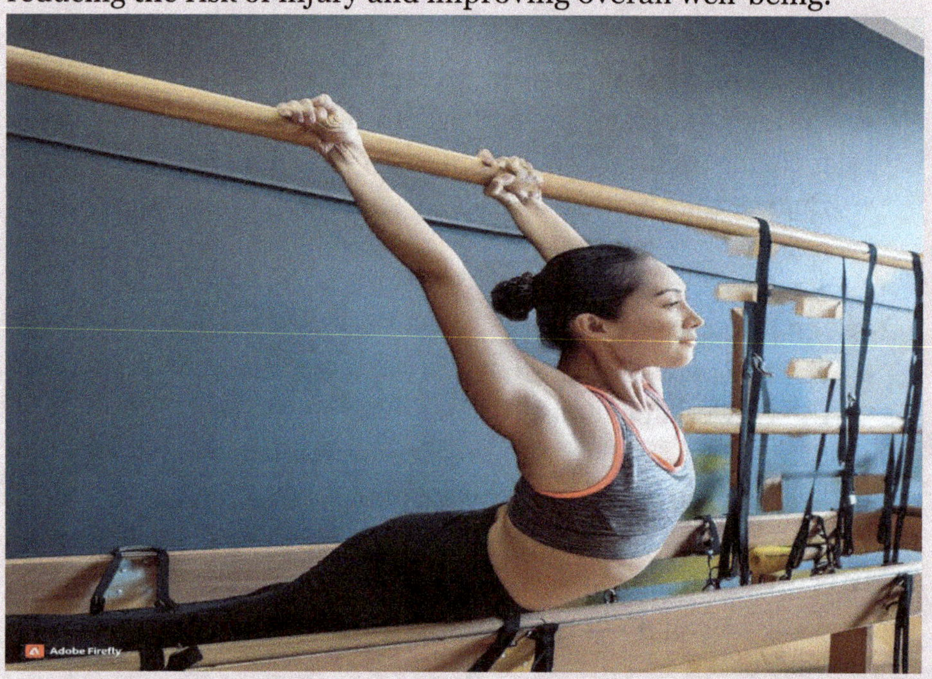

Chapter 3

Setting Up Your Wall Pilates Space

Creating a suitable environment for your Wall Pilates workout is essential to ensure safety and effectiveness. Follow these steps to set up your space:

1. Choose an appropriate wall: Pick a strong wall with a smooth surface that is free from any obstructions or sharp edges.

2. Clear the area: Make sure the surrounding floor space is free from clutter, mats, or any objects that could disrupt your workout.

3. Install a Wall Unit or Anchor Points: Invest in a Wall Pilates unit or install anchor points specifically designed for Wall Pilates. These will securely attach your equipment.

4. Attach Equipment: Set up your Wall Pilates equipment, such as resistance bands, straps, or a wall bar, following the instructions provided by the manufacturer.

5. Add a Mat or Non-Slip Surface: Place a yoga mat or non-slip surface on the floor to provide grip and cushioning.

6. Consider installing a mirror so that you can monitor your form and alignment while exercising.

7. Make sure that the area is well-lit so that you can see your body positioning and movements clearly.

8. Keep water and towels nearby so that you can easily stay hydrated and wipe away sweat.

9. Create a peaceful atmosphere by playing calming music, using aromatherapy, or adding plants to the space.

10. After your workout, make sure to store your equipment properly to keep the area organized and free of clutter.

By following these steps, you will be able to create a Wall Pilates space that is safe, functional, and inviting, enhancing your overall workout experience.

Creating a dedicated workout space

To enhance your Wall Pilates experience and maintain a consistent practice, it is beneficial to create a designated workout area. Consider the following suggestions for creating an ideal space:

1. Allocate a specific area: Set aside a particular room or corner solely for your workout space to establish a clear distinction between exercise and personal time.

2. Natural Lighting: Position your workout area near a window to take advantage of natural light, which can improve your mood and energy levels.

3. Mirrors: Install a mirror to monitor your posture, alignment, and movements during your workouts.

4. Flooring: Opt for a durable and non-slip surface for your workout area, such as a yoga mat, rubber flooring, or a floor specifically designed for Pilates.

5. Keep your Wall Pilates equipment organized and easily accessible by investing in a storage unit or shelves.

6. Enhance your workout experience by installing a sound system for music or guided workouts.

7. Make sure there is good airflow in the room to prevent overheating and discomfort.

8. Maintain a comfortable temperature range (around 68-72°F) to optimize your performance.

9. Minimize distractions by removing or silencing electronic devices to stay focused.

10. Create a peaceful and inspiring atmosphere by adding motivational quotes, plants, or calming artwork.

11. Ensure there is sufficient lighting to see your body positioning and movements.

12. Keep a water bottle and towel nearby for convenience and hydration.

By incorporating these elements, you will create a dedicated workout space that promotes a productive and enjoyable Wall Pilates experience.

Tips for setting up your wall unit and mat

Here are some steps to follow when setting up your Wall Pilates wall unit and mat:

Wall Unit:

1. Choose a comfortable height: Position the wall unit so that the top bar is at a height that feels comfortable for your arms and shoulders.

2. Securely attach it to the wall: Make sure the wall unit is firmly attached to the wall to prevent any movement or falling while using it.

3. Adjust the resistance if possible: If your wall unit has adjustable resistance, start with a lower setting and gradually increase it as you gain strength and endurance.

4. Keep it organized: Store your Wall Pilates equipment, such as straps and handles, in a designated area to maintain an organized and clutter-free workout space.

1. Select the appropriate size: Choose a mat that is big enough to accommodate your body and movements during exercises.

2. Ensure a surface that doesn't slip: Make sure the mat has a surface that prevents slipping and falling while doing exercises.

3. Position it correctly: Place the mat in front of the wall unit, making sure it is centered and aligned with the wall bars.

4. Keep it clean and well-maintained: Regularly clean and take care of your mat to prevent the growth of bacteria and make it last longer.

Additional Tips:

1. Clear the area around: Remove any clutter or obstacles around the wall unit and mat to ensure a safe and effective workout.

2. Use a towel or grip enhancer: Consider using a towel or a product that improves grip on the wall bars to prevent slipping.

3. Start slowly: Begin with slow and controlled movements, gradually increasing your speed and intensity as you become more comfortable with the exercises.

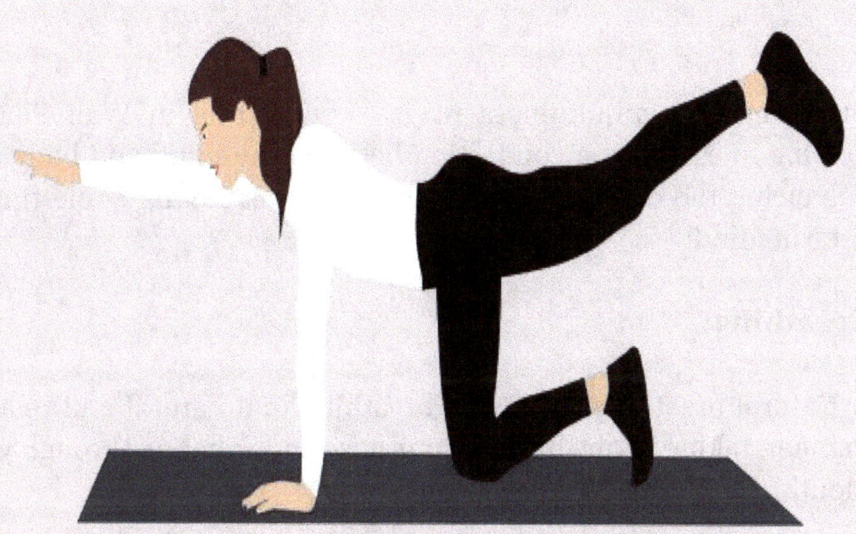

Chapter 4

Breathing and Mindfulness

Breathing and mindfulness play a crucial role in Wall Pilates, helping to establish a connection between the mind and body and enhancing the overall workout experience. Here are some tips to keep in mind:

Breathing:

1. Natural breathing: Focus on breathing in a natural and relaxed manner, taking in air through your nose and exhaling through your mouth.

2. Deep breathing: Take deep breaths, allowing your lungs to fully expand, which can promote relaxation and reduce stress.

3. Synchronized breathing: Coordinate your breath with your movements, inhaling as you expand and exhaling as you contract.

4. Controlled breathing: Maintain a steady and controlled pace of breathing, especially during more challenging exercises.

Mindfulness:

1. Being fully present: Concentrate on the current moment, releasing any distractions and mental clutter.

2. Sensing your body: Develop an awareness of your body's position, alignment, and movements.

3. Proper muscle utilization: Activate the appropriate muscles, avoiding unnecessary tension and strain.

4. Linking the mind and body: Foster a connection between your mind and body, utilizing your breath and movements to unify them.

Additional Suggestions:

1. Begin your workout by practicing mindfulness exercises such as deep breathing or body scanning to help center yourself.

2. Utilize visualization techniques to enhance your mind-body connection by imagining your movements and muscles engaging.

3. Incorporate mindfulness into your daily activities like walking or showering to develop a greater awareness of your mind-body connection.

4. Make breathing and mindfulness a regular part of your daily routine to improve your overall well-being.

By prioritizing breathing and mindfulness, you will have a more comprehensive and efficient Wall Pilates workout, promoting both physical and mental harmony.

The Basic Principles of Breathing

1. Proper breathing promotes efficient oxygenation of the blood, helps maintain focus on tasks, and prevents unnecessary tension, especially in the neck, shoulders, and mid-back. Deep exhalation can also activate the body's deep support muscles.

2. It is recommended to have a three-dimensional breath pattern, expanding the rib cage in all directions without neglecting any areas. During exhalation, the rib cage closes inward and downward while the spine slightly flexes. Therefore, exhaling is suggested to accompany and facilitate spinal flexion.

3. During inhalation, the rib cage opens outward and upward while the spine extends slightly. Therefore, inhaling is suggested to accompany and facilitate spinal extension. Exhaling can also be used during spinal extension to maintain abdominal engagement and support the lumbar spine.

4. It is important to prioritize breath and stability before starting any exercise.

5. Try out different breathing techniques. Lie on your back and observe your natural breath pattern. Pay attention to any specific area, like the abdomen, upper chest, or sides and back of the rib cage, that may be more affected than others.

6. When hugging your knees, sit on a mat with your upper body and head rounded forward. Rest your hands on your knees or shins and keep your neck relaxed.

7. Focus on directing your breath into your entire rib cage, allowing your abdomen to slightly expand. Avoid taking shallow breaths only into your upper chest and shoulders.

8. To help with this breathing pattern, feel the lower posterior-lateral rib cage and encourage full expansion. Engage your abdominal wall lightly, allowing the diaphragm to depress and the abdomen to expand slightly.

9. Engaging the abdominal wall is important for supporting the internal organs and assisting in expelling air from the body. The

transversus abdominis muscle plays a significant role in this process.

By contracting the deep pelvic floor muscles, the transversus can also be activated. It is recommended to incorporate the activation of these stabilizing muscles into the breathing pattern.

10. To feel the contraction and lifting of the pelvic floor muscles, one can try sitting or being on all fours. To feel the activation of the transversus, lie in a neutral position and place fingertips just inside the anterior superior iliac spine. On an exhale, perform a submaximal contraction of the transversus, feeling it tighten beneath the fingers.

11. During this contraction, there may be a sensation of flattening along with a submaximal contraction of the pelvic floor. It is important to avoid hollowing or pulling the belly button towards the spine, and there should be no bulging of muscles beneath the fingers.

12. Regulating the breath by inhaling through the nose and exhaling through the mouth can help achieve a fuller breath pattern. Exhaling through slightly pursed lips can also bring more awareness to the contraction of the abdominal muscles.

while lying on your back

Exhale
Start by gently activating your pelvic floor and transversus muscles. As you exhale deeper, your obliques will also engage to assist in expelling the air.

Inhale

Take a breath in through your nose, while keeping your muscles engaged. Feel the expansion of your rib cage and abdomen in all directions.

The importance of proper breathing in Pilates

Here are some reasons why it is important to breathe properly in Pilates:

- Proper breathing helps activate the specific muscles targeted in each Pilates exercise.
- Deep breathing engages the abdominal muscles, which are crucial for stability and balance.
- Deep breathing prevents shallow chest breathing, which can cause dizziness and lightheadedness.
- Deep breathing helps relax tense muscles in the neck, shoulders, and back.
- Deep breathing strengthens the deep core muscles, which are essential for stability and balance.

Deep breathing can assist in diminishing stress and anxiety by triggering the release of endorphins and decreasing the production of cortisol. It can also aid in relieving tense muscles and preventing muscle strain. Additionally, deep breathing can enhance the oxygen levels in the blood, resulting in increased energy levels and reduced fatigue.

In Pilates, it is important to breathe correctly by inhaling through the nose and exhaling through the mouth. The focus should be on expanding the rib cage in all directions. Additionally, engaging the abdominal and pelvic floor muscles is crucial to support the breath.

It is essential to breathe naturally and smoothly, avoiding holding the breath or shallow breathing. With practice, proper breathing in Pilates can become a habit and enhance the effectiveness of your workout.

Introduction to mindfulness and meditation techniques

Mindfulness and meditation are effective tools for developing awareness, reducing stress, and enhancing overall well-being.

Mindfulness:

- Being fully present in the current moment
- Observing thoughts, emotions, and physical sensations without judgment
- Concentrating on the breath, body, or surroundings

Meditation:

- A practice aimed at cultivating mindfulness
- Focusing on a specific object, thought, or activity
- Quieting the mind and accessing a deeper level of consciousness

Techniques:

1. Body Scan: Either lying down or sitting comfortably, attentively bring attention to each part of the body, starting from the toes and progressing to the head.

2. Mindful Breathing: Concentrate on the breath, experiencing the sensation of air entering and leaving the nostrils.

3. Practice Loving-Kindness Meditation by repeating phrases like "May I experience happiness, may I enjoy good health, may I find peace" to yourself and others.

4. Engage in Walking Meditation by focusing on each step, the sensation of your feet touching the ground, and the movement of your body.

5. Try Guided Meditation by listening to an audio recording that provides instructions and imagery to guide your meditation.

6. Explore Transcendental Meditation by using a mantra to quiet your mind and access a deeper level of consciousness.

7. Incorporate Movement Meditation into your practice by combining physical movement, such as yoga or tai chi, with mindfulness.

8. Utilize Visualization techniques by imagining a peaceful scene or scenario, engaging all your senses to create a mental sanctuary.

Remember, the aim is not to achieve a specific state, but to develop awareness and kindness towards yourself and others. Begin with short sessions (5-10 minutes) and gradually increase the duration as you become more comfortable with the practices.

How to incorporate breathing and mindfulness into your Wall Pilates practice

Incorporating mindful breathing and mindfulness techniques into your Wall Pilates routine can enhance the physical benefits and foster a stronger connection with your body. Here's how you can do it:

1. **Begin by practicing mindful breathing:**
   - Start by focusing your attention on your natural breath, noticing the sensation of the air entering and leaving your nostrils.
   - As you inhale, consciously lengthen your spine and expand your chest.
   - As you exhale, let go of any tension and allow your body to relax.

2. **Coordinate your breath with your movements:**
   - Inhale during expansion and extension movements such as chest expansion and arm reaches.
   - Exhale during contraction and flexion movements like abdominal curls and leg lifts.

3. **Utilize mindful breathing cues:**
   - When inhaling, use the cue "Inhale, lengthen" to remind yourself to lengthen your spine and expand your chest.
   - When exhaling, use the cue "Exhale, release" to prompt the release of tension and relaxation in your body.
   - To synchronize your breath with movement, use the cue "Breathe, move."

4. **Engage in mindful movement:**
   - Concentrate on the sensations you feel in your body while you are in motion.
   - Pay attention to how your core is activated and how your joints move.
   - Take your time and move deliberately, appreciating each moment.

5. **Integrate mindfulness exercises:**
   - Take short breaks during your workout to focus on your breathing and the sensations in your body.

- Practice body scanning, loving-kindness meditation, or guided imagery during periods of rest.

6. **Utilize mindful language:**
- Instead of saying "Push harder," say "Engage your core and lengthen your spine."
- Instead of saying "Try harder," say "Allow your body to move effortlessly and gracefully."

7. **Establish a routine:**
- Start with brief moments of mindfulness and gradually increase them as you become more comfortable with the practice.
- Incorporate mindfulness into your daily schedule, not just during Wall Pilates.

By incorporating mindful breathing and mindfulness into your Wall Pilates routine, you will develop a stronger connection with your body, enhance your physical benefits, and cultivate a greater sense of tranquility and well-being.

Chapter 5

Warm-Up and Preparation

Before beginning your Wall Pilates workout, it is crucial to warm up and prepare your body. Here is a step-by-step guide to help you get ready:

1. **Arrival and Setup (5 minutes):**
   - Arrive at your designated workout area and arrange your Wall Pilates equipment.
   - Wear comfortable clothing and shoes.
   - If desired, play some calming music.

2. **Breathing and Relaxation (5 minutes):**
   - Find a comfortable seated or standing position.
   - Close your eyes and take slow, deep breaths, focusing on the sensation of each breath.
   - While inhaling, elongate your spine; while exhaling, release any tension.
   - Gradually relax your muscles, starting from your toes and working your way up to your head.

3. **Light Cardio (5 minutes):**
   - Engage in gentle cardiovascular exercises, such as marching in one spot, doing jumping jacks, or jogging in one spot. Increase your heart rate and warm up your muscles.

4. **Dynamic Stretching (5 minutes):**

- Proceed to perform dynamic stretches, focusing on swinging your legs, circling your arms, rotating your hips, and twisting your torso. Keep your movements smooth and controlled, preparing your muscles for the upcoming workout.

5. **Wall Pilates Setup (2 minutes):**
- Stand with your feet apart, shoulder-width distance, facing the wall.
- Position your hands on the wall at shoulder height, activating your arms and shoulders.
- Take a deep breath, feeling the connection between your body and the wall.

Now you are prepared to start your Wall Pilates session! Remember to pay attention to your body and adjust the intensity and pace based on your individual needs. Enjoy the fluidity of the exercises!

Dynamic warm-up exercises to prepare your body

Here are some dynamic warm-up exercises that you can do to prepare your body for Wall Pilates:

1. **Leg Swings:**
- Begin by standing with your feet hip-width apart.
- Swing one leg forward and backward, then switch to the other leg.
- Gradually increase the distance and speed of your leg swings.

2. **Arm Circles:**
- Extend your arms straight out to the sides at shoulder height.
- Create small circles with your hands, completing 10-15 repetitions.
- Change directions and repeat the arm circles.

3. **Hip Rotations:**
  - Start by standing with your feet together.
  - Rotate your hips in a large circle, first in a clockwise direction and then in a counterclockwise direction.
  - Repeat this movement for 10-15 repetitions.

4. **Torso Twists:**
  - Stand with your feet shoulder-width apart.
  - Twist your torso to one side, while keeping your feet and hips facing forward.
  - Hold this position for a few seconds, then twist your torso to the other side.

5. Stretch your neck by slowly tilting your head to the side, bringing your ear closer to your shoulder. Hold this position for 10-15 seconds, then switch sides.

6. Perform shoulder rolls by moving your shoulders in a circular motion, first forward and then backward. Repeat this movement for 10-15 repetitions.

7. Extend your wrists by holding your arm straight out in front of you. Lift your hand up and down while keeping your wrist straight. Repeat this exercise for 10-15 repetitions.

8. Rotate your ankles by standing with your feet together. Move your ankles in a circular motion, first clockwise and then counterclockwise. Repeat this rotation for 10-15 repetitions.

9. Lift your knees by standing with your feet together. Bring one knee towards your chest while keeping your foot flexed. Hold this position for a few seconds, then lower your leg and repeat with the other knee.

10. Perform toe taps by standing with your feet together. Lift one foot off the ground and tap your toes in front of the other foot. Repeat this movement on the other side.

Remember to start slowly and gradually increase the intensity and speed as you warm up. These dynamic warm-up exercises will help prepare your muscles and get you ready for your Wall Pilates workout!

Mobility and flexibility exercises for optimal range of motion

Here are some exercises that can help you maintain a good range of motion in your body:

1. Neck Stretch: Gently tilt your head to the side, bringing your ear closer to your shoulder. Hold this position for 30 seconds and then do the same on the other side.

2. Shoulder Rolls: Rotate your shoulders in a circular motion, moving them forward and backward. Repeat this movement for 10-15 times.

3. Chest Expansion: Stand in a doorway and place your hands on the doorframe at shoulder level. Lean forward until you feel a stretch in your chest muscles. Hold this position for 30 seconds.

4. Quad Stretch: Stand with one hand against a wall for support. Bend one knee and bring your foot behind you, holding it with your hand. Hold this stretch for 30 seconds and then switch to the other leg.

5. Perform hip circles by standing with your feet apart and moving your hips in a large circular motion, first in one direction and then

in the opposite direction. Repeat this movement for 10-15 repetitions.

6. To do knee lifts, stand with your feet together and raise one knee towards your chest while keeping your foot flexed. Hold this position for a few seconds, then lower your leg and repeat the movement with the other knee.

7. Stand with your feet apart and perform calf raises by lifting your heels off the ground, raising your calves. Hold this position for a few seconds, then lower your heels back down.

8. Sit on the floor with your legs extended in front of you and lean forward to reach for your toes, stretching your hamstrings. Hold this stretch for 30 seconds.

9. Stand with your feet together and lift one leg straight out to the side, keeping it straight. Hold this position for a few seconds, then lower your leg and repeat the movement with the other leg.

10. Lie on your stomach with your arms extended above your head and slowly lift your arms, shoulders, and upper back off the ground. Hold this position for a few seconds, then lower your upper body back down.

Remember to take deep and slow breaths while holding each stretch to get the maximum benefit. Avoid bouncing or pushing yourself beyond a comfortable range of motion.

Preparing your core and stabilizing muscles

To effectively perform Wall Pilates workouts, it is important to prepare and strengthen your core and stabilizing muscles. Here are some exercises that can help you engage and strengthen these muscles:

1. **Pelvic Floor Activation:**
   - Sit in a comfortable position with your feet on the ground.
   - Activate your pelvic floor muscles by imagining that you are stopping the flow of urine.
   - Hold this contraction for 5 seconds, then release for 5 seconds. Repeat this for 10-15 repetitions.

2. **Transverse Abdominis Activation:**
   - Lie on your back with your knees bent and feet flat on the ground.
   - Activate your transverse abdominis muscle by pulling your belly button towards your spine.
   - Hold this contraction for 5 seconds, then release for 5 seconds. Repeat this for 10-15 repetitions.

3. **Plank:**
   - Begin in a push-up position with your hands shoulder-width apart.
   - Engage your core muscles to support your body.
   - Hold this position for 30-60 seconds, then rest for 30 seconds. Repeat this for 3-5 sets.

4. **Wall Sit:**
   - Stand with your back against a wall and your feet shoulder-width apart.
   - Slowly slide your back down the wall until your thighs are parallel to the floor.
   - Engage your core muscles to support your body.
   - Hold this position for 30-60 seconds, then rest for 30 seconds. Repeat this for 3-5 sets.

5. **Leg Raises:**
   - Lie on your back and stretch your arms out above your head.

- Raise your legs off the floor, keeping them straight.
- Maintain this position for 5 seconds, then lower it for 5 seconds. Repeat this movement for 10-15 repetitions.

6. **Side Plank (each side):**
- Lie on your side with your feet stacked and place your hands under your shoulders.
- Lift your hips off the ground, activating your core muscles.
- Hold this position for 30-60 seconds, then take a 30-second break. Repeat the same exercise on the opposite side.

Remember to breathe naturally and smoothly while engaging your core and stabilizing muscles. Avoid holding your breath or excessively tensing your muscles.

Chapter 6

50 Wall Pilates Workouts for Women

Here are 50 different Wall Pilates workouts specifically designed for women, accompanied by a brief explanation of how to perform each exercise:

1. Wall Push-Ups: Position yourself with your feet shoulder-width apart and place your hands on the wall at shoulder height. Lower your body towards the wall and then push yourself back up.

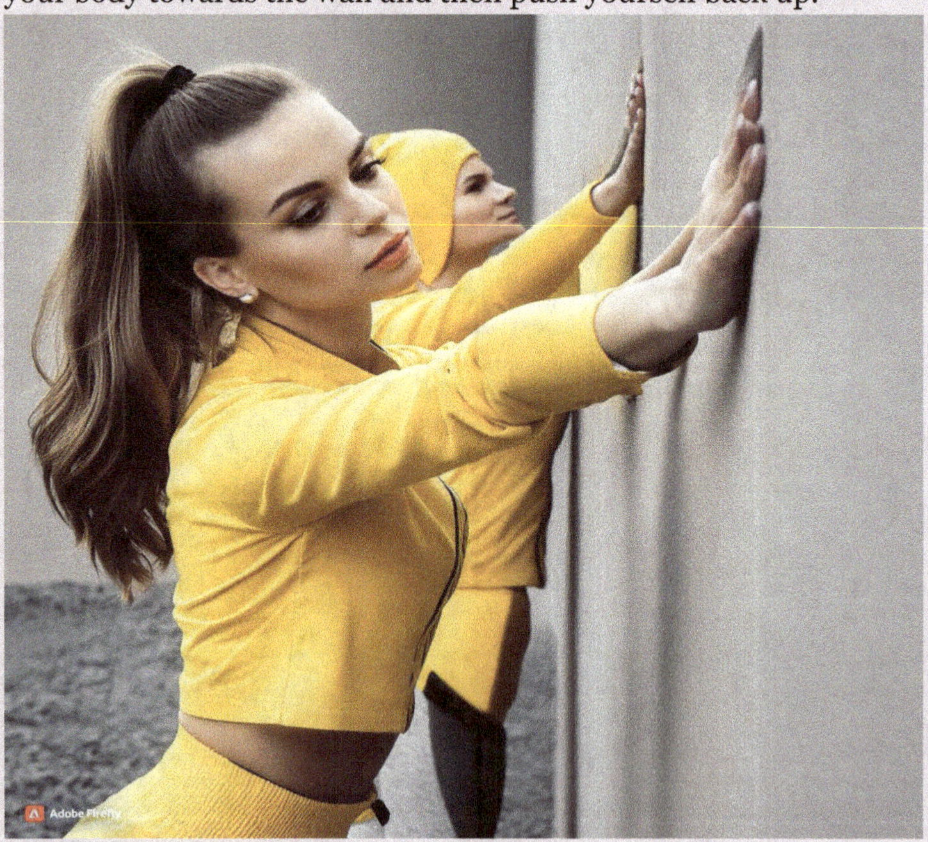

2. Wall Squats: Stand with your feet shoulder-width apart and your back against the wall. Slowly slide down into a squatting position and then stand back up.

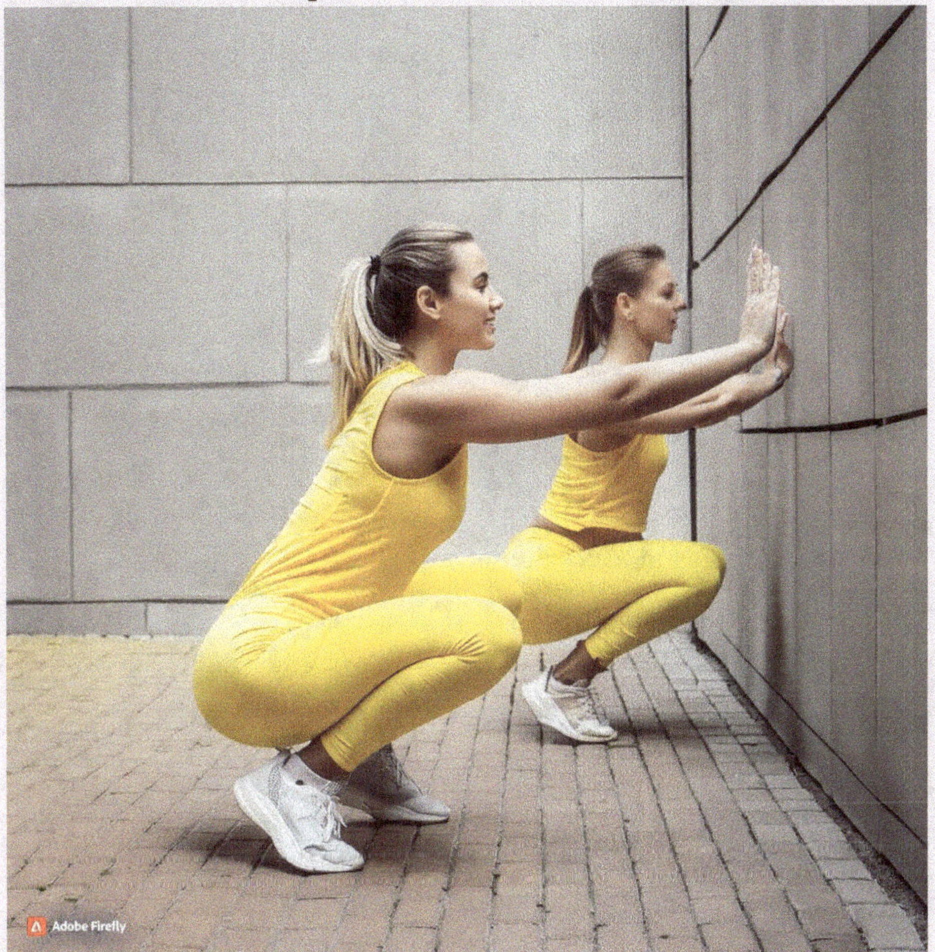

3. Wall Lunges: Stand with your feet together and use one hand on the wall for balance. Take a large step forward with one foot, lower your body down, and then push yourself back up. Alternate between legs.

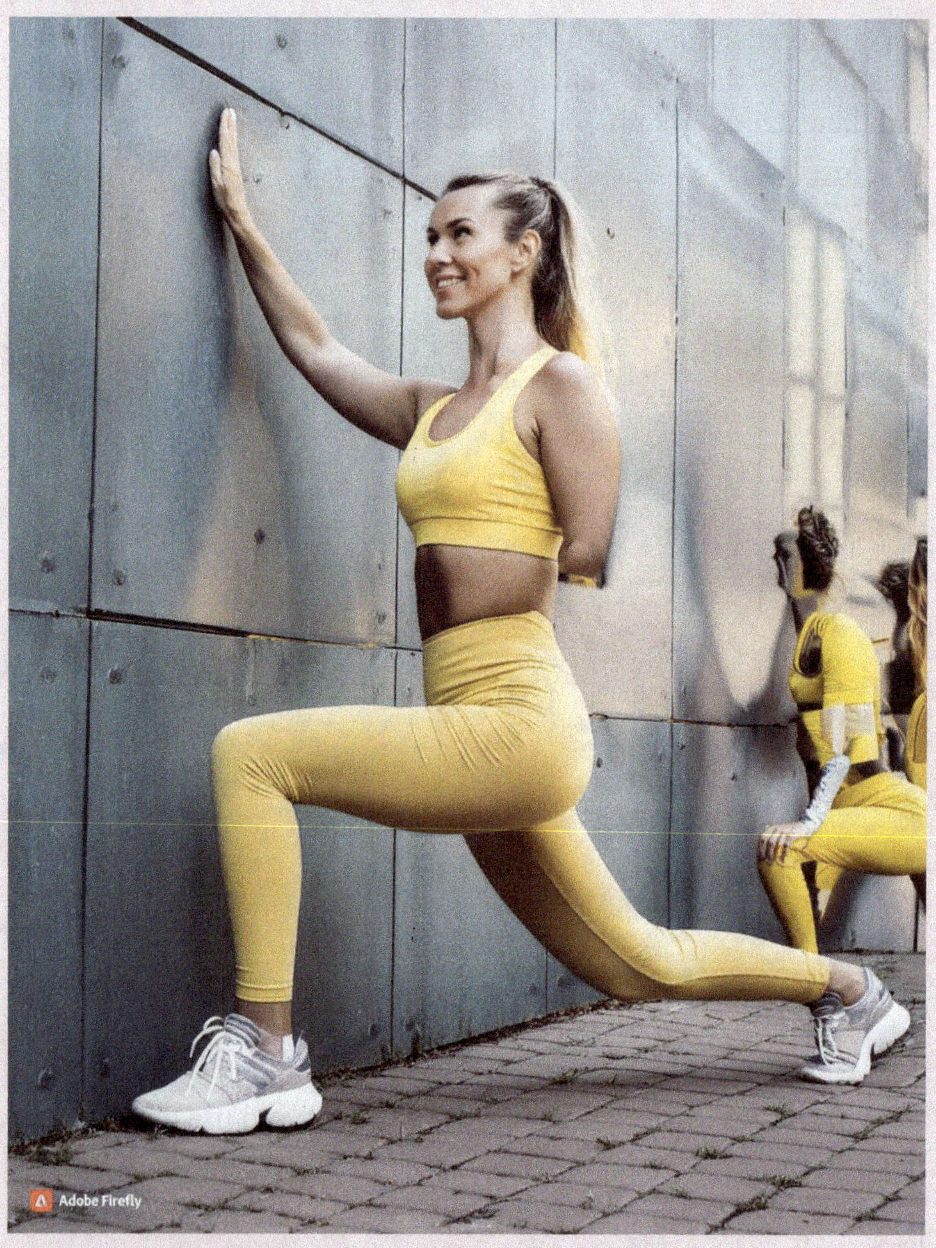

4. Wall Chest Press: Stand with your feet shoulder-width apart and place your hands on the wall at shoulder height. Push your hands against the wall and then release.

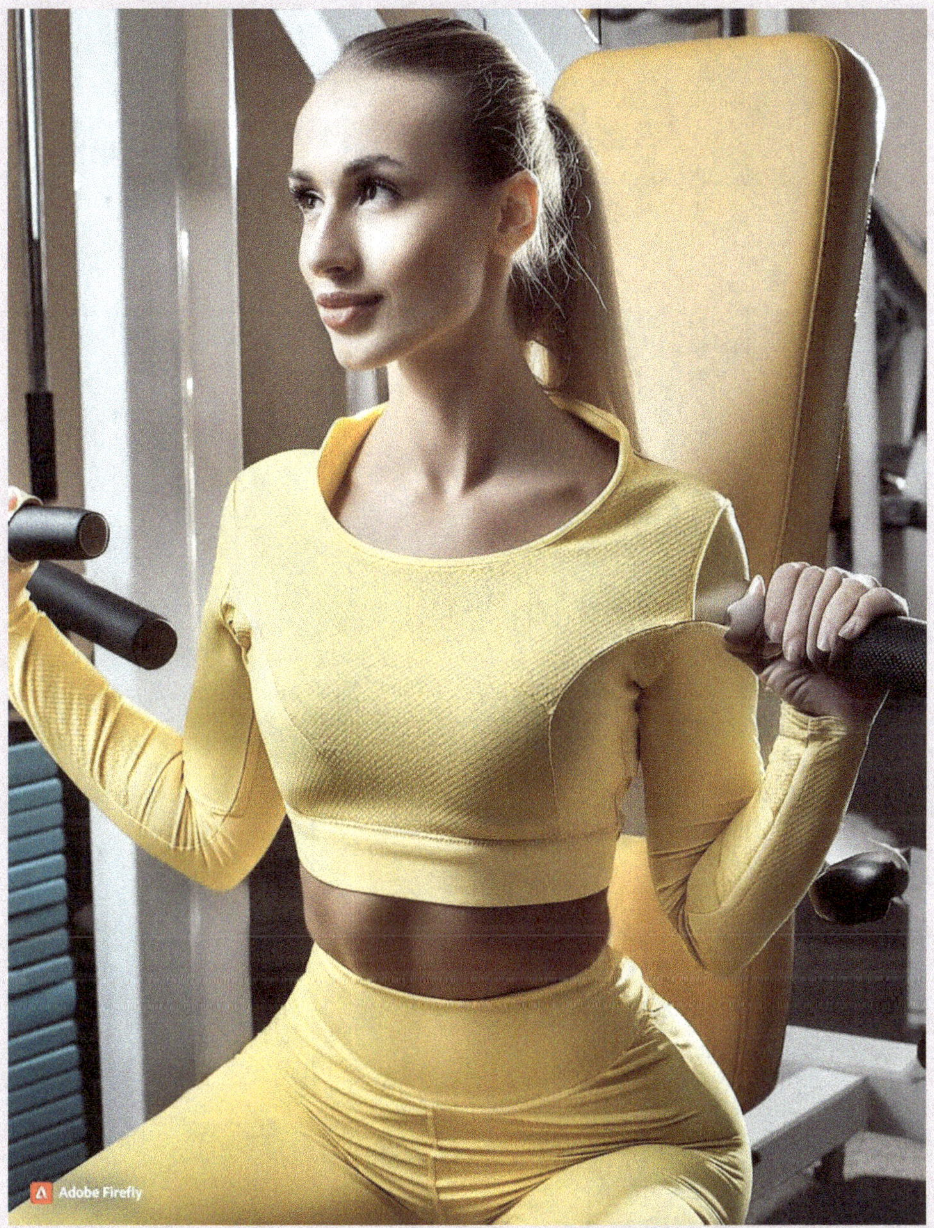

5. Wall Shoulder Rolls: Stand with your feet shoulder-width apart and place your hands on the wall at shoulder height. Roll your shoulders forward and backward in a circular motion.

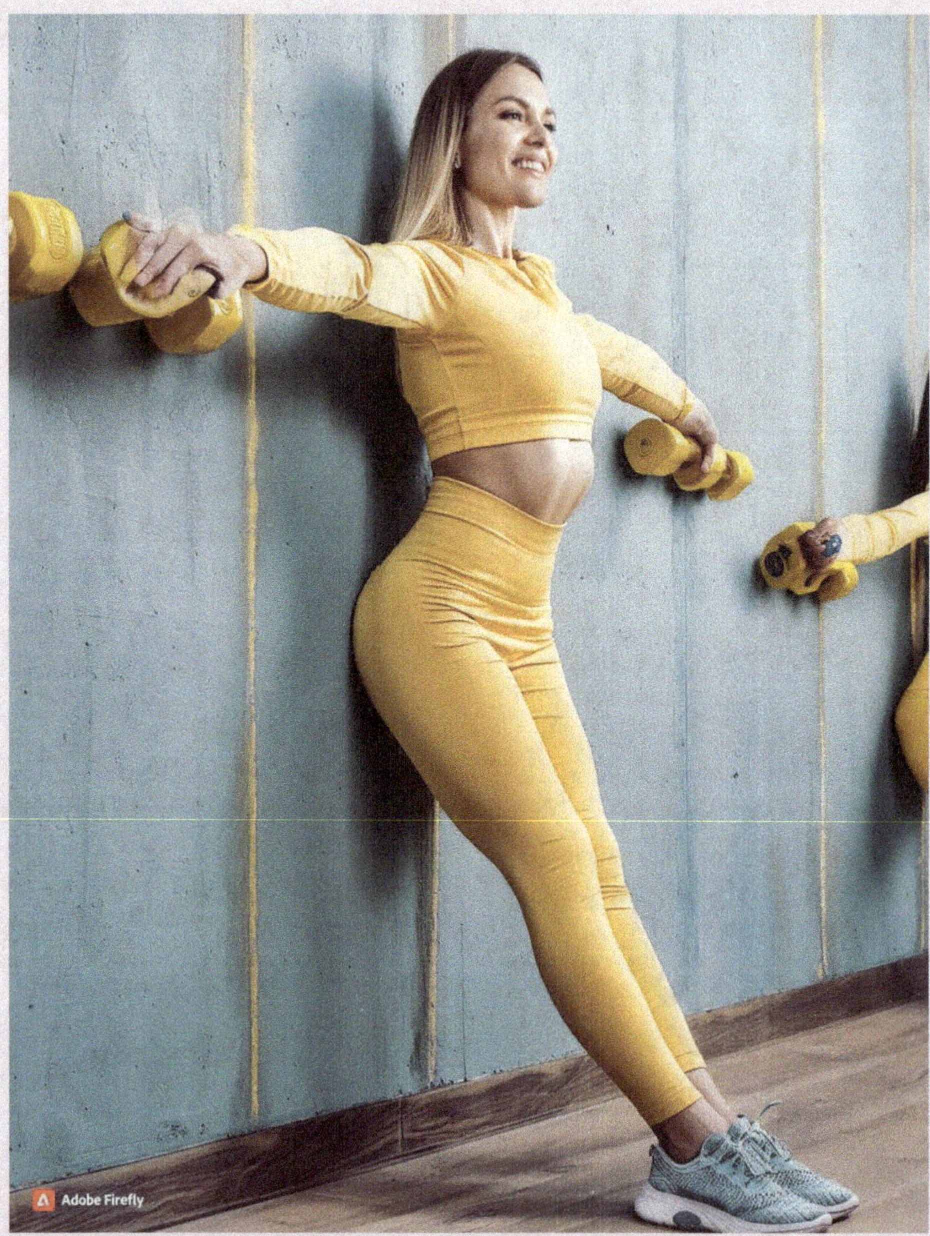

6. Wall Bicep Curls: Stand with your feet shoulder-width apart and place your hands on the wall at shoulder height. Curl your hands up towards your shoulders and then lower them back down.

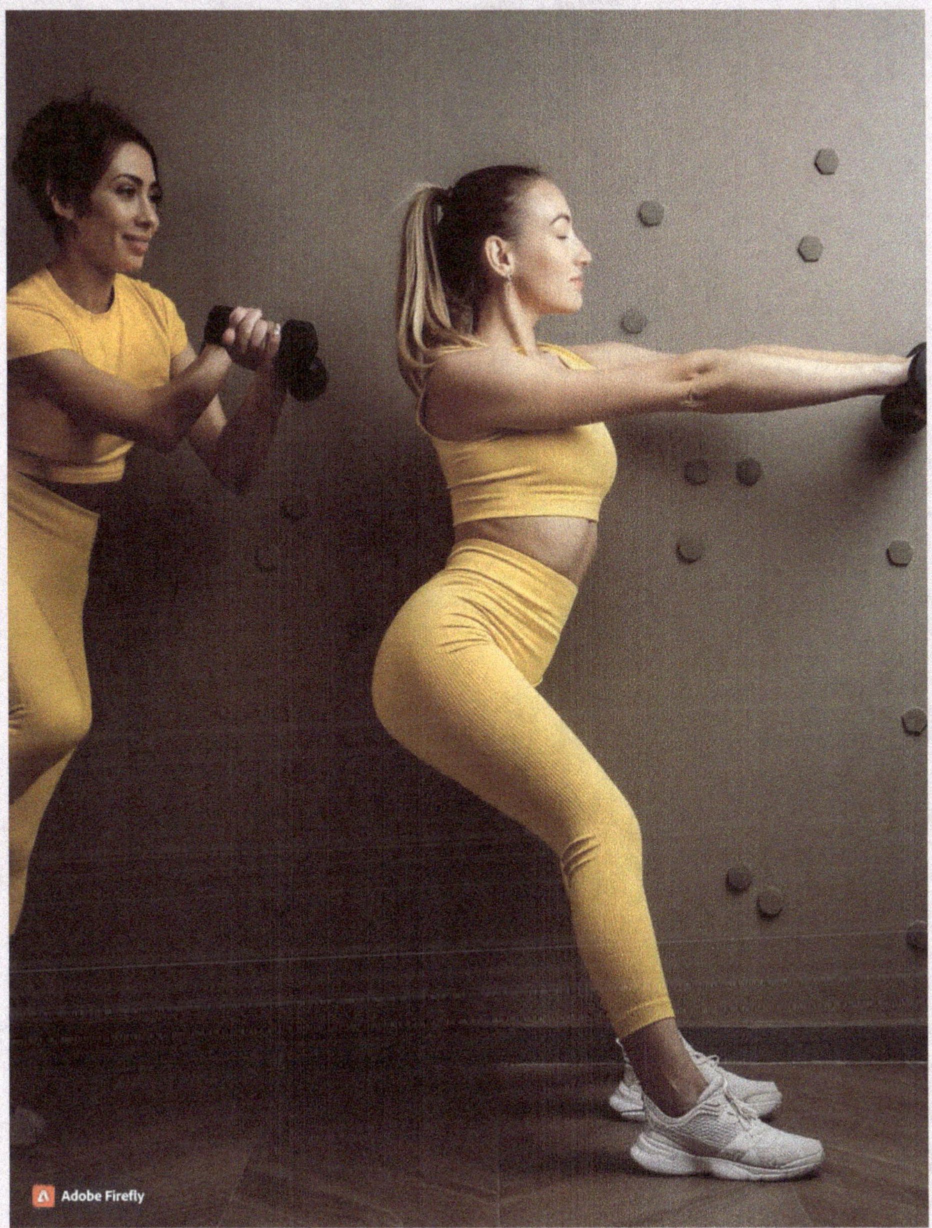

7. Wall Tricep Dips: Stand with your feet shoulder-width apart and place your hands on the wall at shoulder height. Lower your body down by bending your elbows and then straighten your arms.

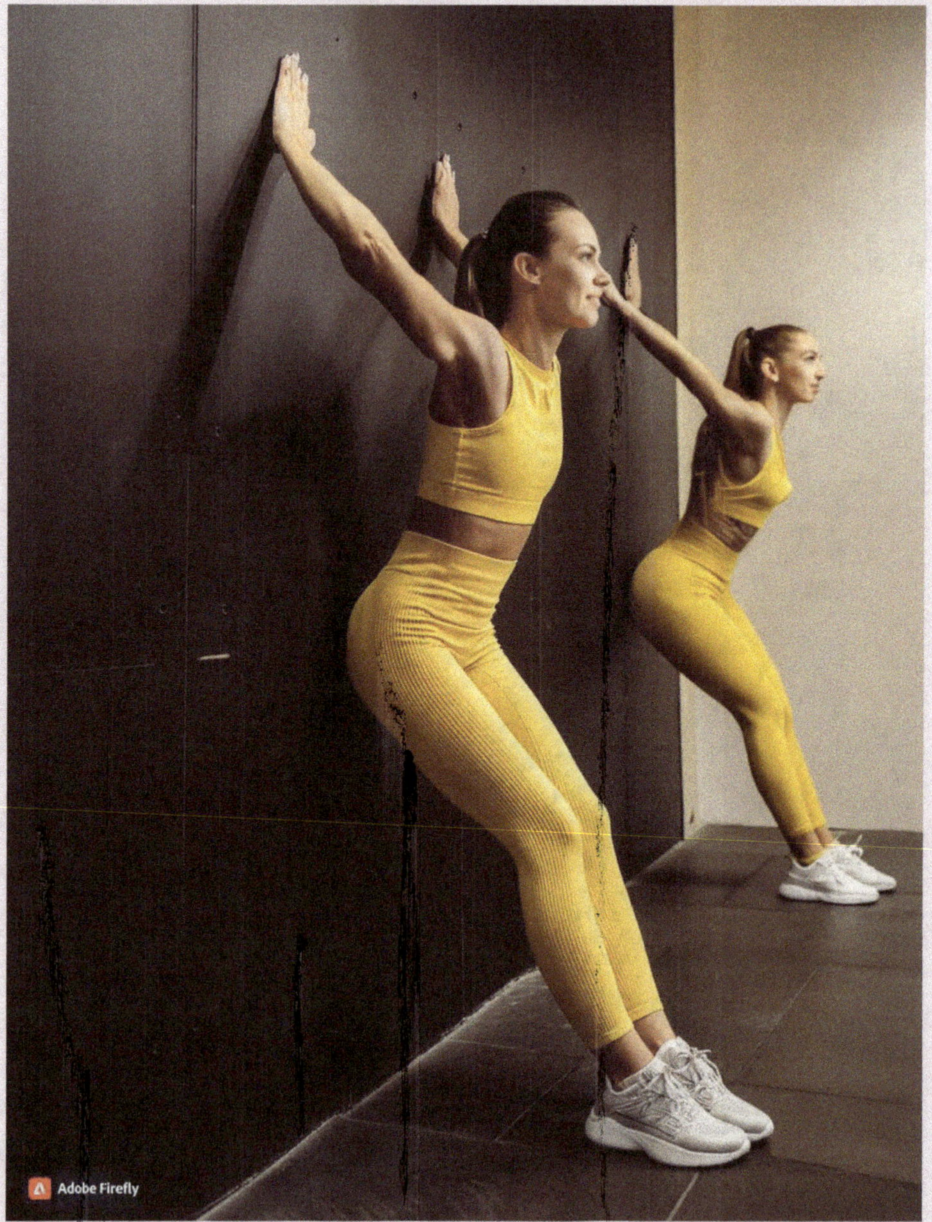

8. Wall Side Bends: Stand with your feet together and place your hands on the wall at shoulder height. Bend your body to one side while keeping your arms straight, then return to the center. Repeat

the   same   movement   on   the   other   side.

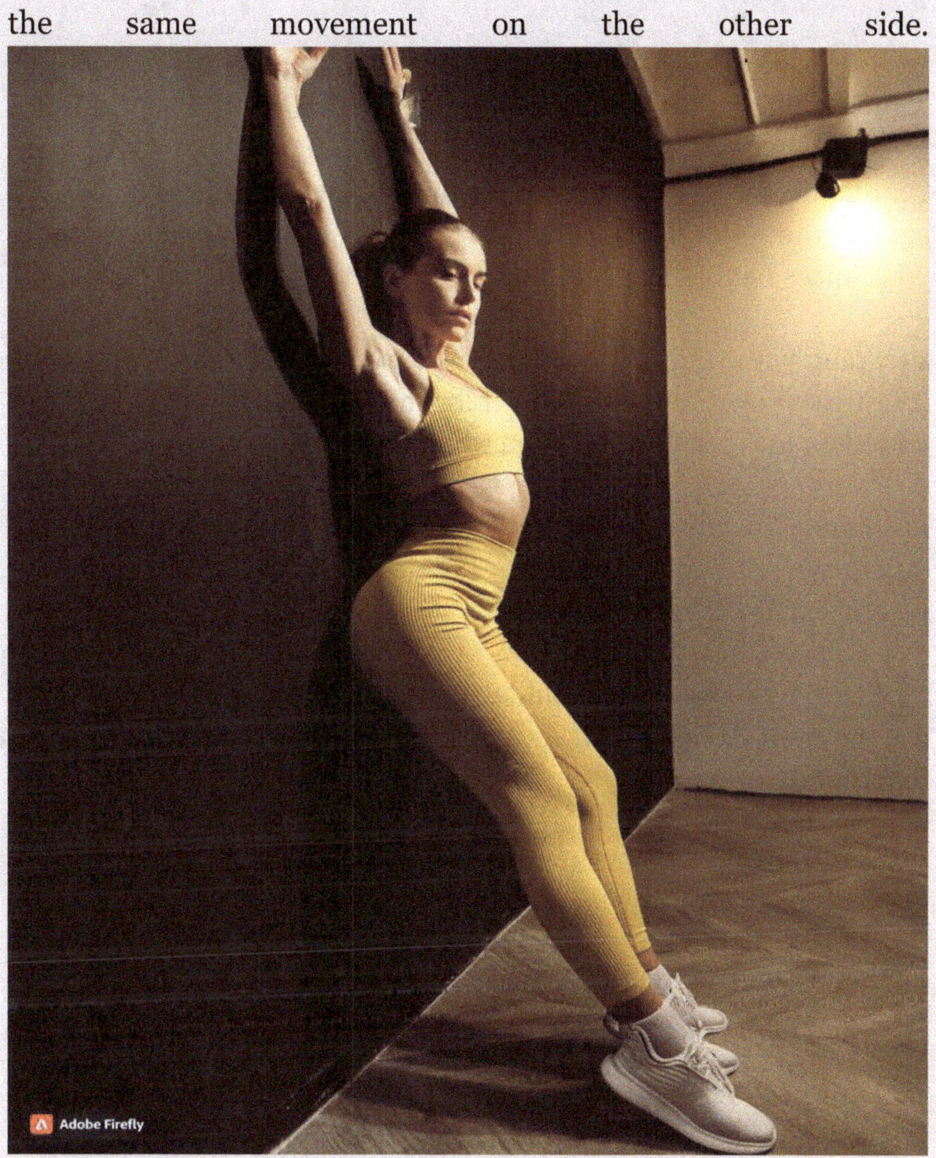

9. Stand with your feet together and place your hands on the wall at shoulder height. Lift one leg out to the side while keeping it straight, then lower it. Switch legs and repeat.

10. Stand with your feet shoulder-width apart and place your hands on the wall at shoulder height. Lift your heels off the ground to raise your calves, then lower them.

11. Begin in a push-up position with your hands on the wall at shoulder height. Engage your core muscles and hold this position.

12. Stand with your feet shoulder-width apart and lean your back against the wall. Slowly slide down into a seated position, keeping your knees bent at a 90-degree angle.

13. Stand with your feet shoulder-width apart and place your hands on the wall at shoulder height. Lift one leg straight out in front of you, then lower it. Switch legs and repeat.

14. Stand with your feet shoulder-width apart and place your hands on the wall at shoulder height. Take a deep breath in, expanding your chest, and then exhale.

15. Stand with your feet shoulder-width apart and place your hands on the wall at shoulder height. Squeeze your shoulder blades together, then release.

16. Stand with your feet shoulder-width apart and place your hands on the wall at shoulder height. Arch your back and look up towards the ceiling, then round your spine and tuck your chin to your chest.

17. Stand with your feet shoulder-width apart and place your hands on the wall at shoulder height. Bend forward at the hips, reaching for your toes, and then straighten back up.

18. Stand with your feet together and place your hands on the wall at shoulder height. Take a large step forward with one foot while keeping your knee straight. Then, bend the front knee and lean forward. Switch legs and repeat.

19. Stand with your feet shoulder-width apart and place your hands on the wall at shoulder height. Bend one knee and keep your foot behind you, then straighten the knee. Alternate legs and repeat.

20. Stand with your feet together and place your hands on the wall at shoulder height. Lift one leg straight out to the side, then lower it. Switch legs and repeat.

21. Stand with your feet shoulder-width apart and place your hands on the wall at shoulder height. Move your hands in small circles for 10 repetitions.

22. Stand with your feet shoulder-width apart and place your hands on the wall at shoulder height. Walk your hands up the wall while keeping your feet shoulder-width apart, then walk back down.

23. Stand with your feet shoulder-width apart and place your hands on the wall at shoulder height. Lift one foot off the ground and tap the heel in front of the other foot. Alternate between legs.

24. Stand with your feet shoulder-width apart and place your hands on the wall at shoulder height. Lift one foot off the ground and tap your toes in front of the other foot. Alternate between legs.

25. Stand with your feet shoulder-width apart and place your hands on the wall at shoulder height. Rotate your ankles in a circular motion, first clockwise and then counterclockwise.

26. Stand with your feet together and place your hands on the wall at shoulder height. Lift one knee towards your chest and then lower it. Alternate legs.

27. Stand with your feet shoulder-width apart and place your hands on the wall at shoulder height. Lift one leg straight out in front of you and then lower it. Alternate legs.

28. Stand with your feet shoulder-width apart and place your hands on the wall at shoulder height. Lift one leg out to the side while keeping it bent, and then lower it. Alternate legs.

29. Stand with your feet together and place your hands on the wall at shoulder height. Bend to one side while lifting the opposite leg.

30. Stand with your feet shoulder-width apart and place your hands on the wall at shoulder height. Press your hands against the wall and lift one leg off the ground, then lower it.

31. Stand with your feet shoulder-width apart and place your hands on the wall at shoulder height. Roll your shoulders forward and backward in a circular motion while lifting one arm off the wall.

32. Stand with your feet shoulder-width apart and place your hands on the wall at shoulder height. Bring your hands up towards your shoulders, while lifting one leg off the ground. Then, lower your hands and leg back down.

33. Stand with your feet shoulder-width apart and place your hands on the wall at shoulder height. Bend your elbows to lower your body down, while lifting one leg off the ground. Then, straighten your arms.

34. Stand with your feet together and place your hands on the wall at shoulder height. Lift one leg straight out to the side, while keeping it straight, and extend the opposite arm. Then, lower your leg and arm.

35. Stand with your feet shoulder-width apart and place your hands on the wall at shoulder height. Lift your heels off the ground to raise your calves, while lifting one arm off the wall. Then, lower your heels and arms.

36. Start in a push-up position with your hands on the wall at shoulder height. Engage your core and lift one leg off the ground, holding the position.

37. Stand with your feet shoulder-width apart and lean your back against the wall. Slowly slide down into a seated position, keeping your knees bent at a 90-degree angle, and extend your arms out to the sides.

38. Stand with your feet shoulder-width apart and place your hands on the wall at shoulder height. Lift one leg straight out in front of you, while lifting the opposite arm off the wall. Then, lower your leg and arm.

39. Stand with your feet shoulder-width apart and place your hands on the wall at shoulder height. Inhale deeply, expand your chest and then extend your arms out to the sides. Exhale.

40. Stand with your feet shoulder-width apart and place your hands on the wall at shoulder height. Squeeze your shoulder blades together and lift one arm off the wall. Then release.

41. Stand with your feet shoulder-width apart and place your hands on the wall at shoulder height. Arch your back, looking up at the ceiling, and extend your arms out to the sides. Then round your spine and tuck your chin to your chest.

42. Stand with your feet shoulder-width apart and place your hands on the wall at shoulder height. Bend forward at the hips, reaching for your toes, and lift one arm off the wall. Then straighten.

43. Stand with your feet together and place your hands on the wall at shoulder height. Take a large step forward with one foot, keeping your knee straight, and extend the opposite arm. Then bend the front knee and lean forward.

44. Stand with your feet shoulder-width apart and place your hands on the wall at shoulder height. Bend one knee and lift the opposite arm off the wall, then straighten.

45. Stand with your feet together and place your hands on the wall at shoulder height. Lift one leg out to the side, keeping it straight, and extend the opposite arm. Then lower.

46. Stand with your feet shoulder-width apart and place your hands on the wall at shoulder height. Walk your hands up the wall while keeping your feet shoulder-width apart. Lift one arm off the wall, then walk back down.

47. Stand with your feet shoulder-width apart and place your hands on the wall at shoulder height. Lift one foot off the ground and tap the heel in front of the other foot, while also lifting the opposite arm off the wall. Then, switch sides and repeat.

48. Stand with your feet shoulder-width apart and place your hands on the wall at shoulder height. Lift one foot off the ground and tap your toes in front of the other foot, while also lifting the opposite arm off the wall. Then, switch sides and repeat.

49. Stand with your feet shoulder-width apart and place your hands on the wall at shoulder height. Rotate your ankles in a circular motion, first clockwise and then counterclockwise, while extending your arms out to the sides.

50. Stand with your feet together and place your hands on the wall at shoulder height. Lift one knee toward your chest, while also lifting the opposite arm off the wall. Then, lower your knee and repeat with the other leg.

Always remember to warm up before starting any workout, listen to your body, and modify or rest when necessary. It is also important to focus on maintaining proper form and technique throughout each exercise.

A full-body workout focusing on core strength and confidence

Here is a workout that targets your entire body and focuses on strengthening your core and building confidence:

Warm-up (5 minutes):

Start with some light cardio exercises like jogging or jumping jacks. Then, do dynamic stretches such as leg swings and arm circles.

Circuit 1: Core Strength

1. Hold a plank position for 30 seconds.
2. Do 15 Russian twists.
3. Perform 15 leg raises.
4. Complete 15 bicycle crunches.
5. Finish with 15 woodchoppers.

Circuit 2: Upper Body

1. Do 15 push-ups.
2. Perform 15 bicep curls.
3. Complete 15 tricep dips.
4. Do 15 shoulder presses.
5. Finish with 15 chest flys.

Circuit 3: Lower Body

1. Perform 15 squats.
2. Do 15 lunges on each leg.
3. Complete 15 calf raises.
4. Execute 15 glute bridges.
5. Perform 15 leg presses.

Circuit 4: Core Strength

1. Hold a side plank for 30 seconds on each side.
2. Do 15 repetitions of Superman exercises.
3. Complete 15 reverse crunches.
4. Perform 15 flutter kicks.
5. Execute 15 draw-ins.

Cool-down (5 minutes):

Engage in static stretching, focusing on the major muscle groups.

This workout targets the muscles in your core, including your abs, obliques, and lower back, while also involving your upper and lower body. Remember to listen to your body and adjust the intensity and volume of the workout based on your personal needs and fitness level.

Boosting Confidence:

Focus on your strengths and achievements.
Set realistic goals and celebrate your progress.
Practice positive self-talk and affirmations.
Surround yourself with supportive individuals who encourage and motivate you.
Take care of both your physical and mental well-being.

Remember, confidence comes from within. Believe in yourself and your abilities, and you will be unstoppable!

"Goddess Glow": A workout targeting toning and sculpting for women's trouble spots

Here are some exercise routines that can help you achieve a radiant and toned appearance in areas that women often struggle with.

Full Body Workout: This workout can be done at home without any equipment. It focuses on toning and sculpting the abs, legs, and the entire body.

High-Intensity Interval Workouts: This workout is designed to promote weight loss, muscle growth, or improved endurance.

Quick Home Workouts: Suitable for all fitness levels, this workout aims to aid in weight loss, muscle toning, buttocks shaping, facial toning, and endurance.

Yoga Programs: This workout concentrates on enhancing flexibility and can be easily performed at home.

Dance Workouts: A fun workout that can be done at home, targeting weight loss and endurance.

It is always advisable to consult a healthcare professional before starting any new exercise routine.

"Prenatal Bliss": A gentle and nourishing workout for expectant mothers

Here are some exercises that can be beneficial for pregnant women:

Pelvic Curl:
This exercise helps strengthen the abdominal muscles that provide support to the growing belly. Lie on your back with your knees bent and feet flat on the ground, about hip-width apart. Take a deep breath in and then exhale as you tilt your pelvis, creating an impression of your spine on the floor. Maintain this position as you continue to exhale and gradually lift your spine off the floor, one vertebra at a time until you reach your shoulder blades. Inhale at the top of the movement and then exhale as you slowly lower your body back down, placing each vertebra back onto the floor until you return to your starting position. Aim for 12 to 15 repetitions.

Pelvic Brace:
This exercise involves gently closing the openings of the urethra, vagina, and anus, while also working the lower abdominal muscles. To perform this exercise, lie on your back with your knees bent and feet flat on the ground, about hip-width apart. Position your pelvis and lower back in a neutral position. Take a deep breath in to prepare, then exhale as you perform a Kegel contraction by gently closing the openings. Notice how your lower abdominal muscles engage during this contraction. Slightly draw in the lower abs while performing the Kegel. Inhale, relax the abs and pelvic floor and then exhale to repeat the contraction. Aim for 2 sets of 8 to 15 repetitions, holding for 3 to 5 seconds each, once or twice a day.

Kneeling Pushups:
This exercise focuses on strengthening the core and upper body. Start by lying flat on your stomach, then push up onto your hands and knees, making sure your knees are positioned behind your hips. Engage your abs and slowly lower your chest towards the floor as you inhale. Exhale as you press back up. Begin with 6 to 10 repetitions and gradually increase to 20 to 24 reps.

Squats:
This workout targets and strengthens the muscles in your lower body, such as the quadriceps, glutes, and hamstrings. Position

yourself in front of a couch, facing away from it. Start with your feet slightly wider than the width of your hips. Use the couch as a reference point to maintain proper form. Lower your body as if you were about to sit on the couch, but rise back up just before your thighs touch it. Take 5 seconds to descend and 3 seconds to ascend. Exhale as you squat and inhale as you stand. Complete 2 sets of 15 to 20 repetitions.

Bicep Curls:
This exercise prepares your arms for the repetitive lifting and holding involved in caring for your baby. Hold dumbbells weighing 5 to 10 pounds and stand with your feet slightly wider than your hips, with your knees slightly bent. Exhale as you gradually bend your elbows, bringing the dumbbells towards your shoulders. Inhale and slowly lower the weights back down. Take 3 seconds to lift the dumbbells and 5 seconds to lower them. Perform 2 sets of 10 to 15 repetitions.

Incline Pushups:
This workout focuses on the chest, triceps, and shoulders. Stand in front of a ledge or railing and position your hands shoulder-width apart on its surface. Step back, create a straight line with your back, and assume a plank position. Slowly bend your arms, lowering your chest towards the railing or ledge. Extend your arms to return to the initial position. Complete 2 sets of 10 to 12 repetitions.

Plié:
This exercise targets the quadriceps, hamstrings, and glutes while enhancing balance. Stand next to the back of a sturdy chair, with the hand closest to the chair resting on it. Keep your feet parallel and hip-width apart. Engage your core by pulling your belly button up and in, while turning your toes and knees out at a 45-degree angle. Bend your knees, lowering your torso as much as possible while maintaining a straight back. Straighten your legs to go back to the starting position. Repeat for the desired number of repetitions.

Side-Lying Inner and Outer Thigh:
This workout targets the core and inner thighs. Lie on your right side with your head resting on your forearm. Bend your right leg at a 45-degree angle and keep your left leg straight. Place your opposite arm on the floor for stability. Lift your left leg to hip height and repeat for a certain number of repetitions. Then, bend your left knee and place it on top of pillows for support. Straighten your right leg and lift it as high as possible for a certain number of repetitions. Switch sides and repeat the exercise.

Plank:
This exercise focuses on strengthening the core, arms, and back. Get into a position where you are on your hands and feet, with your body in a straight line.

"Body Balance": A workout focusing on stability, flexibility, and overall well-being

"Body Balance" is an excellent workout concept! Here is an example routine:

Warm-up (5 minutes):

Light cardio (such as jogging, jumping jacks, etc.)
Dynamic stretching (such as leg swings, arm circles, etc.)

Stability Exercises (20 minutes):

1. Perform single-leg squats (10 repetitions per leg).
2. Walk heel-to-toe (10 steps forward and backward).
3. Hold balance poses (such as tree pose, eagle pose, etc.) for 30 seconds each.

4. Do plank variations (such as side plank, inverted plank, etc.) for 30 seconds each.
5. Utilize a BOSU ball for training (such as single-leg squats, balance poses, etc.) with 10 repetitions per exercise.

Flexibility Exercises (20 minutes):

1. Stretch the hamstrings for 30 seconds per leg.
2. Stretch the hip flexors for 30 seconds per leg.
3. Perform chest stretches for 30 seconds per arm.
4. Roll the shoulders for 10 repetitions.
5. Stretch the quadriceps for 30 seconds per leg.

Well-being Exercises (20 minutes):

1. Practice deep breathing exercises for 5 minutes.
2. Engage in progressive muscle relaxation for 5 minutes.
3. Perform mindful movements (such as tai chi, qigong, etc.) for 10 repetitions.
4. Utilize visualization techniques for 5 minutes.
5. Conclude with a final relaxation period of 5 minutes.

Cool-down (5 minutes):

- Perform static stretching, focusing on major muscle groups.

- Remember to pay attention to your body and adjust the intensity and duration of the workout according to your individual needs and fitness level. It is also crucial to incorporate proper warm-ups and cool-downs to prevent injuries and promote recovery.

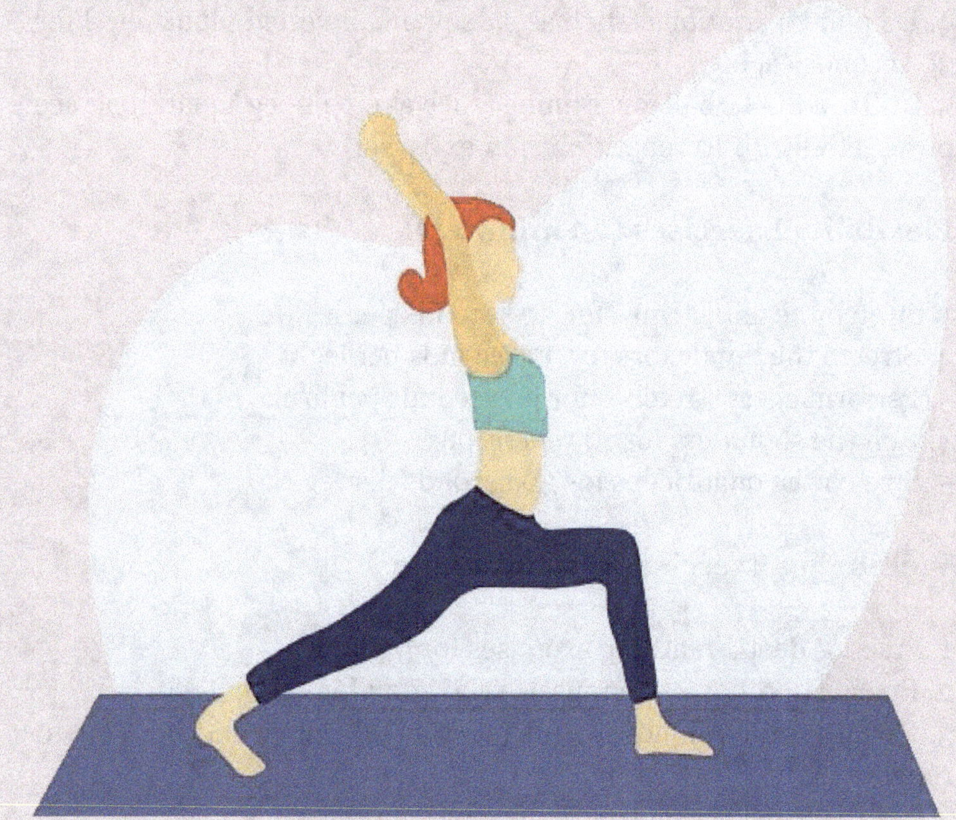

Chapter 7

Modifying and Progressing

Modifications and advancements are crucial concepts in exercise programming. Here's how to implement them:

Modifications:

- Lower the intensity or volume of the workout for beginners or individuals who require a less strenuous option.
- Substitute exercises that have similar movements or target the same muscles.
- Decrease the weight, number of repetitions, or sets.
- Increase the rest time between exercises or sets.

Advancements:

- Increase the intensity or volume of the workout for advanced individuals or those seeking a greater challenge.
- Add weight, repetitions, or sets.
- Decrease the rest time between exercises or sets.
- Introduce new exercises that are more difficult or complex.
- Incorporate progressive overload by gradually increasing the weight or resistance.

Always remember to evaluate individual needs and allow them to advance at their speed. It is important to find a balance between challenge and safety to prevent injuries or exhaustion.

Here are some examples of how to modify and advance exercises:

Squats:
- Modification: Bodyweight squats, sumo squats, or partial squats
- Advancement: Goblet squats, pistol squats, or squat jumps

Lunges:
- Modification: Stationary lunges or assisted lunges
- Advancement: Walking lunges, plyometric lunges, or lunges on one leg

Push-ups:
- Modification: Knee push-ups or incline push-ups
- Advancement: Decline push-ups, diamond push-ups, or push-ups with claps or rotations

Remember that proper form and technique are essential when modifying or advancing exercises. Make sure you or your clients maintain correct alignment and movement patterns to avoid injury.

How to modify exercises for different fitness levels

It is important to modify Wall Pilates exercises for different fitness levels to ensure a safe and effective workout for women. Here's how you can adapt Wall Pilates exercises for different fitness levels:

Modifications for Beginners:

1. Decrease the number of repetitions or sets.
2. Use a lower resistance band or no band at all.
3. Focus on controlled and slow movements.

4. Substitute exercises with simpler movements, such as doing a wall sit instead of a wall squat.
5. Shorten the duration of the workout.

Modifications for Intermediate Level:

1. Increase the number of repetitions or sets.
2. Use a medium resistance band.
3. Incorporate more dynamic movements, like leg lifts and arm circles.
4. Introduce more challenging exercises, such as wall planks and wall bridges.
5. Extend the duration of the workout.

Advanced Modifications:

1. Increase the level of difficulty by using a stronger resistance band or adding weights.
2. Incorporate more challenging movements such as single-leg squats and balance exercises.
3. Amp up the speed and intensity of the exercises.
4. Introduce advanced exercises like wall handstands and wall walks.
5. Extend the duration and intensity of the workout.

Additional Tips:

1. Pay attention to maintaining proper form and technique.
2. Engage your core and maintain control throughout the exercises.
3. Utilize the wall for support and balance when necessary.
4. Listen to your body and take breaks when needed.
5. Gradually increase the intensity and difficulty as you progress.

Examples of modified Wall Pilates exercises:

Wall Squat:
- Beginner: Sit against the wall with knees bent at a 90-degree angle.
- Intermediate: Perform a wall squat with a medium resistance band.
- Advanced: Do a wall squat with a high resistance band and lift one leg.

Wall Push-Up:
- Beginner: Perform a push-up against the wall with knees on the ground.
- Intermediate: Do a push-up against the wall with your eyes on the ground.
- Advanced: Perform wall push-ups with claps or leg lifts.
-
- Always prioritize proper form and technique, and adjust the modifications according to individual fitness levels and needs.

Progressing to more challenging variations

Here are some general suggestions for advancing to more difficult versions of Wall Pilates exercises:

1. Enhance the resistance: Utilize a resistance band with greater tension or incorporate weights into your routine.
2. Alter the angle: Experiment with exercises performed at various angles, such as incline or decline, to provide a fresh challenge for your muscles.

3. Incorporate movement: Introduce dynamic movements like leg lifts or arm circles to intensify the workout.

4. Prioritize control: Emphasize precise movements and maintain control throughout the exercises.

5. Extend the duration: Lengthen the duration of your workout or increase the number of sets and repetitions.

6. To make your workout more difficult, try doing exercises on one side of your body at a time.

7. Use small balls, BOSU balls, or stability balls to add instability and challenge your core.

8. For a greater challenge, try doing wall handstands, wall walks, or wall balances.

9. Increase the intensity by adding explosive movements or quick contractions.

10. Focus on exercises that simulate everyday activities, like squats or lunges, to improve functional strength.

Always prioritize proper form and technique, and gradually move on to more difficult variations as you gain strength, control, and confidence. It's also important to listen to your body and adjust the exercises based on your individual needs and limitations.

Incorporating props and resistance bands for added intensity

Including props and resistance bands in your Wall Pilates workout can increase the difficulty and engage your muscles in different ways. Here are some suggestions for using props and resistance bands:

Props:

1. Small balls: Position a small ball between your back and the wall to provide extra support and challenge during exercises like wall squats and lunges.
2. BOSU ball: Utilize a BOSU ball to introduce instability and challenge your core while performing exercises such as wall planks and wall squats.
3. Stability ball: Incorporate a stability ball to create resistance and challenge your muscles during exercises like wall chest presses and wall rows.
4. Foam roller: Employ a foam roller to add resistance and challenge your muscles during exercises like wall leg raises and wall arm circles.

Resistance Bands:

1. Leg curls: Attach a resistance band to add resistance to your leg curls, targeting your hamstrings and glutes.

2. Chest presses: Apply a resistance band to add resistance to your chest presses, focusing on your chest and shoulders.

3. Rows: Secure a resistance band to add resistance to your rows, targeting your back and arms.

4. To target your shoulder and arm muscles, use a resistance band during your shoulder rotations to provide added resistance.

5. During your leg raises, use a resistance band to add resistance and focus on your core and leg muscles.

Tips for using props and resistance bands:

1. Begin with a lighter resistance and gradually increase it as you gain strength and endurance.
2. Pay attention to maintaining proper form and technique, even when using added resistance.
3. Utilize props and resistance bands to specifically target different muscle groups and add variety to your workout.
4. Experiment with various props and resistance bands to determine which ones work best for you.
5. Remember to breathe and engage your core throughout each exercise.

By incorporating props and resistance bands into your Wall Pilates routine, you can increase the intensity, challenge your muscles in new ways, and elevate your workout to a higher level.

Chapter 8

Common Challenges and Solutions

Here are some typical issues and remedies for Wall Pilates workouts:

Issues:

1. Limited room or equipment availability
2. Trouble with correct posture and technique
3. Restricted range of motion or flexibility
4. Not enough difficulty or intensity
5. Challenges in activating core muscles
6. Difficulty in maintaining proper alignment
7. Time constraints or scheduling limitations
8. Problems in adapting exercises to individual requirements
9. Inadequate support or guidance
10. Stagnation or lack of improvement.

Solutions:

1. Utilize a resistance band or perform bodyweight exercises as alternatives to modify the exercises.

2. Concentrate on maintaining correct posture and technique, and utilize a mirror or record yourself on video to ensure proper form.

3. Begin with modified exercises and progressively enhance the intensity and extent of movement.

4. Increase the difficulty and intensity by adding props or resistance bands.

5. Activate the core muscles by pulling the belly button towards the spine and maintaining proper alignment.

6. Utilize a wall anchor or resistance band to assist in maintaining proper alignment.

7. Arrange shorter workout sessions or utilize online resources for quick workouts.

8. Seek guidance from a certified instructor or use online resources for modifications and direction.

9. Employ progressive overload and vary exercises to avoid reaching a plateau.

10. Include active recovery and stretching to maintain progress and prevent injuries.

Remember, Wall Pilates is a versatile and adaptable workout method that can be adjusted to meet individual needs and challenges. With creativity, patience, and perseverance, you can overcome common obstacles and achieve your fitness goals.

Addressing common issues like back pain, sciatica, and shoulder tension

Wall Pilates can be adjusted to target common problems such as back pain, sciatica, and shoulder tension. Here are some suggestions:

Back Pain:

1. Concentrate on engaging and stabilizing the core.
2. Perform gentle and controlled movements.
3. Avoid excessive arching or twisting.
4. Utilize the wall for support during exercises like wall squats and lunges.
5. Incorporate exercises like wall bridges and wall leg raises to enhance the strength of the back muscles.

Sciatica:

1. Perform gentle and controlled movements.
2. Steer clear of deep lunges or squats.
3. Emphasize exercises that strengthen the glutes and hamstrings.
4. Try exercises like wall leg raises and wall calf raises.
5. Utilize the wall for support during exercises like wall squats and lunges.

Shoulder Tension:

1. Focus on doing exercises that make your shoulder muscles stronger.
2. Move your body gently and in a controlled way.
3. Avoid using heavy weights or resistance.
4. Try doing exercises like making circles with your arms against a wall and rolling your shoulders against a wall.
5. Use a wall for support when doing exercises like push-ups against a wall and chest presses against a wall.

Additional Tips:

1. Pay attention to your body and stop if you feel any pain.
2. Talk to a healthcare professional or a certified Pilates instructor for advice.
3. Make sure to use the correct form and technique.

4. Start slowly and gradually increase how hard and how long you exercise.

5. Include stretching and using a foam roller to complement your workout.

Remember, Wall Pilates is a flexible and gentle workout method that can be adjusted to fit your individual needs and limitations. By addressing common problems and using the right form and technique, you can have a safe and effective workout.

Modifications for injuries or limitations

Here are some adjustments for injuries or limitations specifically for a Wall Pilates workout for women:

1. **Injuries to the Lower Back:**
   - Avoid excessive bending backward or twisting
   - Keep the core muscles engaged and maintain a straight spine
   - Modify leg lifts and circles to minimize strain on the lower back

2. **Injuries to the Knees:**
   - Avoid deep squats or lunges against the wall
   - Use smaller movements and apply gentle pressure
   - Replace wall squats with wall sits or leg raises

3. **Injuries to the Shoulders:**
   - Avoid heavy movements or using weights for the arms
   - Focus on gentle shoulder rotations and squeezing the shoulder blades together
   - Adjust arm circles and movements to reduce strain

4. **Injuries to the Wrists or Hands:**

- Avoid exercises that involve gripping or putting weight on the hands
- Use wrist supports or make modifications (for example, using a resistance band instead of hand weights)

5. Pregnancy or Postpartum:
- Avoid deep twisting movements and bending forward
- Focus on gentle exercises and pelvic floor exercises that are not too intense
- Adjust exercises to accommodate your growing belly and changes in your body

6. Chronic Conditions (e.g., Arthritis, Fibromyalgia):
- Start slowly and gradually increase the intensity of your exercises
- Focus on gentle movements and exercises that are not too harsh on your body
- Use heat or cold therapy to manage any pain or inflammation you may have

7. Mobility or Balance Limitations:
- Use a wall for support and to help with balance
- Focus on exercises that can be done while seated or standing with the support of a wall
- Gradually increase the range of motion and challenges to your balance

Here are some specific modifications for Wall Pilates exercises:

Wall squats: Do not go too low, keep your back against the wall, and engage your core muscles

Wall push-ups: Use your knees for support instead of your toes, or try wall chest presses instead

Wall leg raises: Lift your legs only a few inches off the ground, and avoid using heavy weights or resistance

Remember to consult with a healthcare professional or fitness expert to determine the best modifications for your specific injury or limitation.

Troubleshooting common mistakes and plateaus

Here are some suggestions for addressing common errors and reaching a plateau in Wall Pilates:

Common Errors:

1. Incorrect Technique: Ensure that you maintain correct posture, activate your core muscles, and perform controlled movements.
2. Inadequate Warm-up: Always warm up before beginning your workout to prevent injuries and prepare your muscles.
3. Excessive Strain: Pay attention to your body's signals and take regular breaks to prevent fatigue and overcome plateaus.
4. Irregular Practice: Strive to practice Wall Pilates consistently, ideally 2-3 times a week, to achieve steady progress.

Plateaus can be overcome by gradually increasing the intensity, weight, or reps of your exercises to challenge your muscles. It is also important to incorporate stretching exercises to improve flexibility and range of motion. To prevent muscle imbalance, focus on exercises that target opposing muscle groups. Mental fatigue can be avoided by mixing up your routine, trying new exercises, or working out with a partner to stay motivated.

To troubleshoot plateaus, analyze your form by recording yourself or working with a trainer to identify and correct any issues.

Changing your routine by trying new exercises, modifying existing ones, or using different equipment can also help challenge your muscles. Focus on the mind-muscle connection by engaging your core, focusing on controlled movements, and connecting with the muscles you're targeting. Taking breaks and allowing your muscles time to rest and recover is important to avoid fatigue and prevent plateaus. Consistency, patience, and self-awareness are key to overcoming common mistakes and plateaus in Wall Pilates.

Chapter 9

Integrating Wall Pilates into Your Lifestyle

Here are some suggestions for incorporating Wall Pilates into your everyday life:

1. Make it a priority: Treat Wall Pilates as an essential part of your daily or weekly schedule, similar to brushing your teeth or showering.

2. Begin with small steps: Start with shorter sessions (20-30 minutes) and gradually increase the length and frequency as your body becomes more accustomed to it.

3. Find a peaceful area: Locate a quiet and comfortable space in your home or workplace where you can practice Wall Pilates without any distractions.

4. Invest in a reliable wall anchor: It is crucial to have a sturdy wall anchor to ensure the safety and effectiveness of your Wall Pilates exercises.

5. Utilize online resources: Follow Wall Pilates YouTube channels, blogs, or social media accounts to find inspiration, tutorials, and motivation for your workouts.

6. Add variety: Combine Wall Pilates with other exercises or activities such as cardio, yoga, or strength training to create a well-rounded fitness routine.

7. Establish a routine: Make Wall Pilates a part of your daily schedule, whether it's right after waking up or before going to bed, to ensure it becomes a sustainable habit.

8. Find a workout partner: Practice Wall Pilates with a friend, family member, or coworker to stay motivated and hold each other accountable.

9. Monitor your progress: Take photos, measurements, or keep track of your workouts to track your progress and stay motivated.

10. Stay consistent: Aim to practice Wall Pilates at least 2-3 times a week, ideally at the same time each week, to see steady progress and make it a lasting lifestyle habit.

Remember, integrating Wall Pilates into your life is a journey, and consistency is crucial. Start small, be patient, and celebrate your achievements along the way!

How to incorporate Wall Pilates into your daily routine

Here are some suggestions on how to include Wall Pilates in your daily schedule:

1. Morning Warm-up: Begin your day by dedicating 10-15 minutes to a Wall Pilates session. This will enhance blood circulation, and flexibility, and boost your energy levels.

2. Lunch Break Workout: Utilize your lunch break to squeeze in a quick 20-30 minute Wall Pilates session. This will rejuvenate and re-energize you for the rest of the day.

3. Post-Work Routine: After finishing work, unwind with a 30-40 minute Wall Pilates session. This will help alleviate stress and tension accumulated throughout the day.

4. Before Bed Stretch: Conclude your day with a 10-15 minute Wall Pilates stretching session. This will promote relaxation and prepare your body for a restful sleep.

5. Replace Commercial Breaks: Instead of remaining sedentary during TV commercial breaks, engage in a few Wall Pilates exercises to stay active and involved.

6. Utilize the time you spend waiting for things like coffee or appointments to do a quick 5-10-minute session of Wall Pilates.

7. During your daily commute, make use of the time by incorporating Wall Pilates exercises while waiting for public transportation or during a bus/train ride.

8. If you have a job that requires sitting at a desk for long periods, take regular breaks to do Wall Pilates exercises and reduce the amount of time you spend being sedentary.

9. Make fitness a fun and bonding experience by involving your kids or partner in Wall Pilates exercises during family time.

10. Establish a specific time of day that works for you and make it a habit to consistently incorporate Wall Pilates into your daily routine.

Remember, even small amounts of Wall Pilates practice can have a positive impact on your physical and mental well-being!

One month Wall Pilates workout Routine

Here is a one-month Wall Pilates workout routine, with a focus on a different muscle group each day:

Week 1

Monday (Chest and Shoulders):
- Wall push-ups (3 sets of 10 reps)
- Wall chest press (3 sets of 10 reps)
- Wall shoulder rolls (3 sets of 10 reps)

Tuesday (Lower Body):
- Wall squats (3 sets of 10 reps)
- Wall lunges (3 sets of 10 reps per leg)
- Wall calf raises (3 sets of 15 reps)

Wednesday (Core):
- Wall plank (3 sets of 30-second hold)
- Wall bicycle crunches (3 sets of 10 reps)
- Wall leg raises (3 sets of 10 reps)

Thursday (Back and Biceps):
- Wall rows (3 sets of 10 reps)
- Wall bicep curls (3 sets of 10 reps)
- Wall shoulder blade squeezes (3 sets of 10 reps)

Friday (Lower Body):
- Wall squats with leg lift (3 sets of 10 reps)
- Wall side lunges (3 sets of 10 reps per leg)
- Wall glute bridges (3 sets of 10 reps)

Week 2

Monday (Chest and Shoulders):
- Wall push-ups with claps (3 sets of 10 reps)
- Wall chest flys (3 sets of 10 reps)
- Wall shoulder rotations (3 sets of 10 reps)

Tuesday (Lower Body):
- Wall squats with calf raise (3 sets of 10 reps)
- Wall curtsy lunges (3 sets of 10 reps per leg)
- Wall side leg lifts (3 sets of 10 reps)

Wednesday (Core):
- Wall plank with arm raise (3 sets of 30-second hold)
- Wall Russian twists (3 sets of 10 reps)
- Wall teasers (3 sets of 10 reps)

Thursday (Back and Biceps):
- Wall rows with rotation (3 sets of 10 reps)
- Wall bicep curls with rotation (3 sets of 10 reps)
- Wall shoulder blade squeezes with rotation (3 sets of 10 reps)

Friday (Lower Body):
- Wall squats with leg lift and calf raise (3 sets of 10 reps)
- Wall side lunges with leg lift (3 sets of 10 reps per leg)
- Wall glute bridges with leg lift (3 sets of 10 reps)

Week 3

Monday (Chest and Shoulders):
- Wall push-ups with rotation (3 sets of 10 reps)
- Wall chest press with rotation (3 sets of 10 reps)
- Wall shoulder rotations (3 sets of 10 reps)

Tuesday (Lower Body):
- Wall squats with calf raise and leg lift (3 sets of 10 reps)
- Wall curtsy lunges with leg lift (3 sets of 10 reps per leg)
- Wall side leg lifts with leg lift (3 sets of 10 reps

Wednesday (Core):
- Wall plank with leg lift and arm raise (3 sets of 30-second hold)
- Wall bicycle crunches with leg lift (3 sets of 10 reps)
- Wall leg raises with rotation (3 sets of 10 reps)

Thursday (Back and Biceps):
- Wall rows with rotation and leg lift (3 sets of 10 reps)
- Wall bicep curls with rotation and leg lift (3 sets of 10 reps)
- Wall shoulder blade squeezes with rotation and leg lift (3 sets of 10 reps)

Friday (Lower Body):
- Wall squats with leg lift, calf raise, and glute bridge (3 sets of 10 reps)
- Wall side lunges with leg lift and glute bridge (3 sets of 10 reps per leg)
- Wall glute bridges with leg lift and calf raise (3 sets of 10 reps)

Week 4

Monday (Chest and Shoulders):
- Wall push-ups with claps and rotation (3 sets of 10 reps)
- Wall chest flys with rotation (3 sets of 10 reps)
- Wall shoulder rotations with leg lift (3 sets of 10 reps)

Tuesday (Lower Body)

- Wall squats with calf raise, leg lift, and glute bridge (3 sets of 10 reps)
- Wall curtsy lunges with leg lift and glute bridge (3 sets of 10 reps per leg)
- Wall side leg lifts with leg lift and glute bridge (3 sets of 10 reps)

Wednesday (Core):
- Wall plank with leg lift, arm raise, and rotation (3 sets of 30-second hold)

Tips for maintaining motivation and consistency

Here are some suggestions for staying motivated and consistent with your Wall Pilates workout routine:

1. Establish clear and attainable objectives: Clearly define your goals and ensure they are specific, measurable, achievable, relevant, and time-bound (SMART).

2. Establish a regular schedule: Create a consistent routine that includes specific times of the day, durations, and frequencies for your workouts.

3. Diversify your routine: Incorporate variety into your workouts to avoid monotony and prevent reaching a plateau.

4. Monitor your progress: Keep a workout log or utilize a fitness app to track your advancements, including the exercises performed, sets and repetitions completed, and weights used.

5. Having a workout partner can be a great source of motivation and accountability.

6. Give yourself small rewards when you reach milestones or complete a certain number of workouts.

7. Find ways to incorporate Wall Pilates into your daily routine, like doing quick workouts during TV commercial breaks.

8. Remember that the benefits of Wall Pilates go beyond just physical appearance and focus on how it improves your overall health and well-being.

9. Don't be too hard on yourself if you miss a workout or don't see immediate results. Progress takes time and everyone has off days.

10. Stay motivated and inspired by following fitness influencers, reading motivational stories, or looking at before-and-after photos.

11. Make Wall Pilates a regular part of your routine, like brushing your teeth or taking a shower.

12. Consider working with a certified Pilates instructor or personal trainer to stay motivated and accountable.

Remember, consistency and motivation are like muscles that need regular exercise to grow stronger. With time and effort, you can establish a consistent routine and stay motivated to achieve your fitness goals.

Combining Wall Pilates with other forms of exercise and self-care

Combining Wall Pilates with other forms of exercise and self-care can boost your overall fitness and well-being. Here are some suggestions for integrating Wall Pilates with other activities:

1. **Yoga or stretching**: Enhance your flexibility and balance by incorporating Wall Pilates into your yoga or stretching routine.
2. Cardiovascular exercises: Improve your heart health by adding activities such as running, cycling, or swimming to your workout regimen.

3. **Strength training**: Build muscle and increase your overall strength by including exercises like weightlifting or resistance band workouts alongside Wall Pilates.

4. **High-intensity interval training (HIIT)**: Challenge yourself with a full-body workout by combining Wall Pilates with HIIT sessions.

5. **Mind-body exercises**: Enhance mental clarity and reduce stress by combining Wall Pilates with practices like meditation, deep breathing, or tai chi.

6. To enhance your cardiovascular health and connect with nature, consider incorporating walking or hiking into your daily routine.

7. For a comprehensive workout that is gentle on the body, try combining Wall Pilates with swimming or water exercises.

8. If you're looking for a joint-friendly cardiovascular workout, consider adding cycling or spinning to your exercise routine.

9. For a lively and energetic full-body workout, combine Wall Pilates with dance-based workouts like Zumba or hip hop.

10. Improve your mental and emotional well-being by including self-care activities such as journaling, reading, or taking relaxing baths in your daily routine.

Here are some tips for integrating Wall Pilates with other exercises and self-care practices:

- Start gradually to avoid exhaustion.
- Pay attention to your body's needs and rest when necessary.
- Choose activities that bring you joy and make you feel good.
- Treat your workouts and self-care routines as important appointments.
- Keep your routine diverse to prevent boredom and plateaus.

Remember, combining Wall Pilates with other exercises and self-care practices is an excellent way to prioritize your overall health and well-being.

Chapter 10

Conclusion and Next Steps

Congratulations on completing the Wall Pilates workout routine! You have taken a significant step towards improving both your physical and mental health. Here are some important reminders:

- Pay attention to your body and take breaks when necessary.
- Stay hydrated and maintain a balanced diet to fuel your body.
- Vary your exercise routine to avoid getting bored and to prevent reaching a plateau.
- Set new goals and challenges for yourself to keep progressing.
- Keep prioritizing self-care and your mental well-being.

Here are the next steps to consider:

- Explore other types of exercise and self-care activities that can complement your Wall Pilates routine.
- Think about working with a certified Pilates instructor or personal trainer who can provide personalized guidance.
- Share your progress and inspire others to start their fitness journey.
- Keep track of your progress and celebrate your achievements along the way.

Remember, fitness is a continuous journey, not a final destination. Stay committed, stay consistent, and most importantly, stay true to yourself. You can do it!

Summary of main points or important lessons learned

This is a brief overview of the key takeaways and valuable insights gathered from our discussion on Wall Pilates:

Key Takeaways:

1. Wall Pilates is a variation of Pilates that utilizes a wall for both support and resistance.

2. It is particularly beneficial for beginners or individuals requiring modifications.

3. Wall Pilates can enhance flexibility, balance, strength, and overall physical fitness.

4. Additionally, it serves as an effective method to alleviate stress and enhance mental well-being.

5. Consistency and motivation play crucial roles in witnessing progress and attaining objectives.

Important Lessons Learned:

1. Begin at a slow pace and gradually increase the intensity and duration of your workouts.

2. Pay attention to maintaining proper form and engaging your core muscles.

3. Vary your exercise routine to avoid getting bored and to prevent hitting a plateau.

4. Listen to your body and take breaks when necessary.

5. Incorporate Wall Pilates with other types of exercise and self-care activities for a well-rounded fitness regimen.

6. Give equal importance to self-care and mental well-being alongside physical fitness.

7. If needed, seek guidance from a certified Pilates instructor or personal trainer.

8. Keep track of your progress and celebrate your achievements along the way.

Remember, the most crucial aspect is to find a fitness routine that suits you and that you enjoy. Consistency and motivation are essential for reaching your goals!

Encouragement to continue your Wall Pilates journey

As you continue on your journey, remember that progress may not always be straightforward. Some days you will feel motivated and strong, while other days you will have to overcome challenges. But that's alright! It's all part of the process.

Always remember why you started: to improve your physical and mental well-being, to feel more confident and empowered, and to take care of yourself. Keep those reasons in mind and let them inspire you to keep going.

You have the ability to achieve anything you set your mind to. Don't be too hard on yourself if you miss a workout or don't see immediate results. Instead, focus on the progress you have already made and celebrate your small victories.

Continue pushing forward, even when things get difficult. Because beyond those challenges lies a stronger, healthier, and happier version of yourself. And that is worth fighting for.

So, keep showing up, keep working hard, and keep smiling. You are doing this, and you are succeeding!

Resources for further learning and growth.

eBooks: There is a wide selection of eBooks available on Pilates for people of all skill levels. "Everything Pilates" and "Caged Lion: Joseph Pilates and His Legacy" are excellent options for beginners and those interested in delving deeper into the history of Pilates.

Podcasts: Podcasts such as "Pilates Unfiltered" and "The Pilates Goddess Podcast" offer a great opportunity to learn more about Pilates culture from industry experts and community teachers.

Apps: Pilates apps are ideal for individuals who live far from their preferred Pilates studios or feel intimidated and want to start learning independently. These apps provide essential instructional content and have user-friendly interfaces. Some apps even offer access to live virtual classes with teachers and instructors.

Videos: Many content creators regularly upload instructional videos for Pilates. If you are just starting, it can be helpful to search for beginner-friendly or low-impact videos. These videos typically engage your entire body and include exercises like Cat and Cows and plank hip twists to leave you feeling energized and confident throughout the day.

For additional resources, you can also explore ACE | Health and Fitness Education, Research, and Career Support.

www.ingramcontent.com/pod-product-compliance
Lightning Source LLC
Chambersburg PA
CBHW081524250726

48659CB00009B/2931